Islam and Biomedical Research Ethics

This book is a contribution to the nascent discourse on global health and biomedical research ethics involving Muslim populations and Islamic contexts. It presents a rich sociological account about the ways in which debates and questions involving Islam within the biomedical research context are negotiated – a perspective which is currently lacking within the broader bioethics literature. The book tackles some key understudied areas, including: the role of faith in moral deliberations within biomedical research ethics; the moral anxiety and frustration experienced by researchers when having to negotiate multiple moral sources and how the marginalisation of women or the prejudice and abuse faced by groups, such as sex workers and those from the LGBT community, are encountered and negotiated in such contexts. The volume provides a valuable resource for researchers and scholars in this area by providing a systematic review of ethical guidelines and a rich case-based account of the ethical issues emerging in biomedical research in contexts where Islam and the religious moral commitments of Muslims are pertinent.

The book will be essential for those conducting research in low- and middle-income countries that have significant Muslim populations and for those in Muslim-minority settings. It will also appeal to researchers and scholars in religious studies, social sciences, philosophy, anthropology and theology, as well as the fields of biomedical ethics, Islamic ethics and global health.

Mehrunisha Suleman is a postdoctoral researcher at the Centre of Islamic Studies, University of Cambridge.

Biomedical Law and Ethics Library

Scientific and clinical advances, social and political developments and the impact of healthcare on our lives raise profound ethical and legal questions. Medical law and ethics have become central to our understanding of these problems, and are important tools for the analysis and resolution of problems – real or imagined.

In this series, scholars at the forefront of biomedical law and ethics contribute to the debates in this area, with accessible, thought-provoking, and sometimes controversial, ideas. Each book in the series develops an independent hypothesis and argues cogently for a particular position. One of the major contributions of this series is the extent to which both law and ethics are utilised in the content of the books, and the shape of the series itself.

The books in this series are analytical, with a key target audience of lawyers, doctors, nurses, and the intelligent lay public.

Series Editor: Sheila A. M. McLean

Professor Sheila A.M. McLean is Professor Emerita of Law and Ethics in Medicine, School of Law, University of Glasgow, UK.

Available titles:

Health Research Governance in Africa
Law, Ethics, and Regulation
Cheluchi Onyemelukwe-Onuobia

Revisiting Landmark Cases in Medical Law
Shaun D. Pattinson

Healthcare Ethics, Law and Professionalism
Essays on the Works of Alastair V. Campbell
Edited by Voo Teck Chuan, Richard Huxtable and Nicola Peart

Religion, Medicine and the Law
Clayton Ó Néill

Islam and Biomedical Research Ethics
Mehrunisha Suleman

For more information about this series, please visit: www. routledge.com/Biomedical-Law-and-Ethics-Library/book-series/CAV5

Islam and Biomedical Research Ethics

Mehrunisha Suleman

Routledge
Taylor & Francis Group

LONDON AND NEW YORK

First published 2021
by Routledge
2 Park Square, Milton Park, Abingdon, Oxon OX14 4RN

and by Routledge
605 Third Avenue, New York, NY 10017

First issued in paperback 2022

Routledge is an imprint of the Taylor & Francis Group, an informa business

© 2021 Mehrunisha Suleman

Publisher's Note
The publisher has gone to great lengths to ensure the quality of this reprint but points out that some imperfections in the original copies may be apparent.

British Library Cataloguing-in-Publication Data
A catalogue record for this book is available from the British Library

Library of Congress Cataloging-in-Publication Data
A catalog record has been requested for this book

ISBN 13: 978-0-367-51387-0 (pbk)
ISBN 13: 978-0-367-19147-4 (hbk)
ISBN 13: 978-0-429-20068-7 (ebk)

DOI: 10.4324/9780429200687

Typeset in Galliard
by Taylor & Francis Books

To all my teachers

"That there is nothing for humankind, except that (good) which they strive for"
— *Quran (The Star, Verse 39)*

"So long as you write what you wish to write, that is all that matters; and whether it matters for ages or only for hours, nobody can say."
— Virginia Woolf, *A Room of One's Own*

Contents

List of illustrations   viii
Foreword   ix
Preface   xi
Acknowledgements   xii
Key Islamic ethico-legal terms   xiv
List of abbreviations   xvi

1   Introduction   1

2   Guideline review: Why is a guideline search and review necessary?   28

3   Role of institutional forms of Islam in biomedical research ethics:
    Religious texts, scholars and their legal edicts   74

4   Islamic responses to the ethical issues of HIV/AIDS: Deeper analysis
    of the role of *ijtihad* and *fatawah* in the context of global health
    research ethics   95

5   Women and biomedical research ethics: Religion, culture and ethics   110

6   Personal faith and biomedical research ethics: Encountering the moral
    universe of Muslim researchers   128

7   Negotiating multiple moral resources: Key findings and
    recommendations for future research   142

8   Methodological annexe   155

Appendix   205
Bibliography   209
Index   220

Illustrations

Figures

1.1   The three levels of the normative sources of Islam and how the different levels interrelate   18

8.1   Diagram of political and religious structures in Malaysia   159

Tables

2.1   Guideline search strategy   30

2.2   Research ethics guidelines found in 21 OIC countries – Guidelines for 18 countries available in English   35

2.3a   Ethical protections stated in 24 documents of 18 OIC Countries   42

2.3b   Ethical protections stated in 24 documents of 18 OIC Countries   45

2.3c   Ethical protections stated in 24 documents of 18 OIC Countries   47

2.4a   Mention of Islam, Islamic sources or the Muslim religio-cultural context in ten documents from eight OIC countries   51

2.4b   Mention of Islam, Islamic sources or the Muslim religio-cultural context in ten documents from eight OIC countries   57

2.4c   Mention of Islam, Islamic sources or the Muslim religio-cultural context in ten documents from eight OIC countries   63

8.1   Malaysia participant profile, including gender (male/female), age, researcher (Y/N), REC member (Y/N), guideline developer (Y/N), Islamic scholar (Y/N), and informal training in the Islamic sciences (Y/N)   177

8.2   Iran participant profile, including gender (male/female), age, researcher (Y/N), REC member (Y/N), guideline developer (Y/N), Islamic scholar (Y/N), informal training in the Islamic sciences (Y/N)   179

8.3   Rationale for the semi-structured interview guide showing themes that were derived from the literature and guidelines   183

8.4   A schematic of the coding framework   188

Foreword

I am delighted to have the opportunity to welcome the publication of this timely and important book, which provides a rich and fascinating analysis of contemporary Islamic medical ethics. Based on in-depth interviews with medical doctors and researchers in several countries, Mehrunisha Suleman reveals the complex and difficult ethical questions arising in the conduct of medical research today and how those questions are understood and engaged with from a Muslim perspective by doctors and researchers in their encounters with patients. This is essential reading for anyone interested in the ethics of medical research or medical practice in the Islamic world, and in the day-to-day lives of Muslim patients and their doctors.

Medical research is increasingly an international endeavour. Much research takes place in countries with significant Muslim populations and is conducted by researchers and doctors who may themselves be Muslim. This book and the research informing it will be of direct relevance to those who conduct, fund, or regulate such research. It will also be of broader interest and relevance to those who are working with Muslim patients or research participants wherever they are in the world.

The book begins with a review and overview of approaches to ethics in Islam. It explains the roles of key texts and how they relate to other important sources of authority. This is both accessible to people who are new to this field and offers an in-depth analysis of key principles and texts that will be of real value to those who are students of ethics. What becomes apparent in this analysis is both the variety of approaches of Islamic ethics, and the subtle and careful ways in which ethical problems in medical research can be addressed. In the book, Mehrunisha Suleman discusses the challenges presented to Islamic ethics by developments in medicine, by the spread of HIV, and by the changing roles of women. She explores ways in which these are being and could be responded to by scholars and practitioners of Islamic medical ethics.

Apart from the impact of technological developments in medicine, and societal change, perhaps the greatest ethical problem facing doctors and medical researchers working in Muslim majority countries is one of how best to make sense in practice of the multiple sources of advice and guidance available to them. In addition to that from the Islamic world mentioned above, international, national, and regional ethics guidelines continue to proliferate. How in practice are doctors and researchers to go about making practical ethical decisions in their day-to-day work with patients and research participants? Little if any work has been previously published exploring the moral worlds of Muslim doctors and those who work with Muslim majority populations. At the heart of this book is a set of chapters reporting on the experiences of individual researchers and doctors in two Muslim-majority countries: Iran and Malaysia. It shows how on a day-to-day basis, those who work in these spaces identify, reflect on, and make ethical judgements in the context of the guidelines and sources of authority mentioned above, but also in the context of their own beliefs and commitments as Muslim doctors or researchers. These chapters provide important insights into the moral worlds and difficult decisions facing those – doctors and researchers – who are working in such situations: their struggles, where they look for solutions and so on.

This is an interesting, timely, and important contribution to the literature on global health ethics. It will be of particular interest and relevance to medical professionals working with Muslim patients, and to anyone involved in the planning or conduct of medical research in international contexts.

Michael Parker
Director of the Wellcome Centre for Ethics and
Humanities and the Ethox Centre
University of Oxford

Preface

This book began from a series of conversations I had almost ten years ago with Professors Tony Hope and Mike Parker at the Rosemary Rue Building in Oxford. Both Tony and Mike inspired my inquisitiveness in ethics, whilst I was a medical student. They both helped to nurture and enable the writing of this volume. Becoming aware of the recent atrocities involving biomedical researchers and physicians in Europe and North America, I began reading and researching about the importance of research governance, safety of participants and populations as well as the role of normative bioethical resources. Classes at the Harvard School of Public Health on Global Health Research Ethics run by Professors Dan Wikler and Richard Cash sparked an interest in how global health research ethics governance can be successfully implemented and sustained with the dizzying number of international guidelines. Whilst simultaneously studying the Islamic sciences, spending time with healthcare professionals and researchers in Zambia and Kenya, I increasingly became aware of the complex moral nexus involved in ethical decision-making in the context of global health research. The latter consisting not only of local and/or international guidelines, but also local cultural and religious norms. These observations led me to consider how bioethics is done in practice and what the role of different moral resources are in contexts where international guidelines are but one source of ethical decision-making. Such questions sparked the design and development of my DPhil research upon which this book is largely based. The aim of this volume is not to settle age-old debates about universalism and relativism, nor is it to define or delineate the role of religion and culture. Rather, it is to contribute to the fields of social science and bioethics by sharing voices and perspectives yet unrepresented in many academic debates relating to biomedical research governance.

Balliol College and the Ethox Centre
University of Oxford, 2019

Acknowledgements

Supervisors

Firstly, I would like to express my heartfelt thanks to Professors Mike Parker and Ray Fitzpatrick for their tireless support, kindness and encouragement during this research.

Academic support

A huge debt and thanks to Professor Abdul Aziz Sachedina and Dr Akram Nadwi for their long-standing teaching and training in the Islamic sciences and ethics, without which my DPhil research and this book would not have been possible. I would also like to acknowledge Dr Aasim Padela for his session on Islamic bioethics that he offered in Cambridge at the Centre for Islam and Medicine.

Special thanks to everyone at the Ethox centre, in particular Prof Tony Hope, Ms Susan Barrington, Ms Mary Foulkes, Ms Jane Beinart, Dr Mikey Dunn, Dr Patricia Kingori, Dr Mark Sheehan, Prof Maureen Kelly, Dr Angeliki Kerasidou and Dr Ruth Horn for their invaluable advice, support and friendship. I would also like to acknowledge the Nuffield Department of Population Health and, in particular, Professor Sasha Shepperd for her kind advice and guidance throughout this research.

Thank you to Dr Ayman Shabana for providing access to the Georgetown University Library in Doha. I am grateful to Ms Erica Ison for her generosity in reading portions of the thesis and overall support of the research. A huge thanks to Professor Martin Burton and everyone at Balliol College for supporting this research and providing me with an intellectual home during my DPhil at Oxford.

A special thanks to Nia Roberts at the Knowledge Centre, University of Oxford, who provided invaluable guidance and support in developing the search strategy, identifying relevant databases and search terms for the literature and guideline review. She also assisted tirelessly in helping me obtain relevant full text references through the inter-library loan system.

Funding

I would like to thank the Medical Research Council and the Nuffield Department of Population Health for funding this research and offering supplementary funding for the fieldwork that was critical for the qualitative study.

Collaborators

A special thanks to Firoz Abdul Hamid, Professor Lokman Saim and Dr Ehsan Shamsi for their enthusiasm and generosity in supporting my field visits in Malaysia and Iran. I would also like to thank all of the respondents who agreed to participate in this study. Their insights have been invaluable in making this research possible and will hopefully contribute to work beyond this study.

Permissions

I would like to thank World Scientific Publishing Co for permission to reproduce parts of the text from my article "Biomedical research ethics in the Islamic context: Reflections on and challenges for Islamic Bioethics," which was chapter 5 in *Islamic Bioethics: Current Issues and Challenges*, edited by A. Bagheri and K. Alali (World Scientific Publishing Co., Singapore, 2017), pp. 197–228.

I would also like to thank Jessica Kingsley Publishers for permission to reproduce parts of the text from my article "Islam, Ethics and Care," which was chapter 1 in *Faith and Ethics in Health and Social Care Improving Practice Through Understanding Diverse Perspectives*, edited by A Gallagher and C Herbert (Jessica Kingsley Publishers, London, 2019), pp. 121–134.

Publishers

I am indebted to Alison Kirk and Emily Summers at Routledge for supporting the publication of this book. Thanks also to the entire Routledge editorial and publishing team as well as the anonymous reviewer for their helpful advice and guidance.

Friends and family

A very special thanks to my parents and entire family for their wisdom, tireless enthusiasm for my work and immeasurable support. And, finally, thanks to Arzoo Ahmed for lending inspiration and friendship throughout this research and beyond.

Key Islamic ethico-legal terms

I have independently translated the terms below directly from Arabic, unless otherwise stated.

Adab	Virtue
Alim	An Islamic scholar who is recognized as an expert in Islamic law and theology (OED online, 2016)
Aql	Reason or rationality
Aqhlaq	Proper conduct
Ash'ari	School of theology, which considers that moral truths, or knowledge of what is good and bad, can only be known from revelation and not by reason alone. This is a popular school amongst Sunni Muslims, who are predominant in Malaysia.
Darabah	Some Islamic scholars say the word means "to hit"; others say it means to "move away"
Dharurah	Necessity
Faqih	A jurist
Fatwah pl. fatawah	Legal edict
Fiqh	Islamic jurisprudence
Fitnah	Temptation (OED online, 2016)
Fitrah	Intuitive nature
Fardh	Compulsory
Hadith	Tradition of the Prophet Muhammad, his sayings, practices and teachings that have been recorded and collated.
Halal	Permissible
Haram	Unlawful
Jama'a	Community of believers
Jizyah	Tax payable by non-Muslims residing in a Muslim state
Ijma	Consensus of scholarly opinion
Ijtihad	Independent reasoning – where a legal opinion is extracted from scriptural sources or independently in the absence of explicit scriptural instruction.
Ilm al Aqhlaq	Science of virtues

Imam	One who leads the prayer
Jizya	Tax
Kalam	Theology
Khalifah	Commander of the believers
Madhab	School of Islamic law
Maqasid	Objectives or goals
Maqasid al Shariah	Objectives of the Shariah
Marja'	One to be followed
Maslaha	Public good or public interest
Mufasirun	Commentators on the *Quran*
Mufti	An Islamic scholar who has the training and expertise in formulating *fatawah* or legal edicts through the process of ijtihad or independent reasoning.
Mu'tazili	School of theology which considers that moral truths or knowledge of good and bad can come from reason and revelation working together. This school was inherited by Shi'i Islam, which is predominant in Iran.
Nushuz	Disobedience
Qiwammah	Authority
Qiyas	Analogical reasoning
Quran	Revelation from God received by the Prophet Muhammad
Shariah	Broadly considered Islamic law, however, many scholars describe it as "the way" or "how to be a Muslim" (Ramadan, 2009, p. 360)
Shia	Partisans of Ali. A sect of Muslims who believe that Ali should have been Muhammad's successor.
Shubahaat	Doubtful matters according to Islamic law
Sunni	Followers of communal tradition. A sect of Muslims who believe that the order of succession from Muhammad was through Abu Bakr, Umar, Uthman and then Ali.
Sunnah	Tradition of the Prophet Muhammad
Ta'ah	Obedience
Tafsir	Quranic exegesis
Tasawwuf	Sufism – "Study of the mystic's path; the respective stages and states of inward journeying towards God" (Ramadan, 2016, p. 11)
Tawhid	Belief in the oneness of God
Urf	Local custom
Wahy	Revelation
Wilayah	Guardianship

List of abbreviations

AD	Anno Domini
AIDS	Acquired immune deficiency
AKU	Aga Khan University
CILE	Research Center for Islamic Legislation and Ethics
CIOMS	Council for International Organisations of Medical Sciences
COHERD	Conference on Health Research for Development
CPR	Cardiopulmonary resuscitation
DNAR	Do not attempt resuscitation
FDA	Food and Drug Administration
GCC	Gulf Cooperation Council
GCP	Good clinical practice
GDP	Gross domestic product
HIV	Human immunodeficiency virus
ICH	International Conference on Harmonisation
IKIM	Institute of Islamic Understanding
IMSE	Islamic Medical and Scientific Ethics
IOMS	Islamic Organisation of Medical Sciences
IRB	Institutional Review Board
IV	Intravenous
IVDU	Intravenous drug user
JAKIM	Ministry of Islamic Development
LGBT	Lesbian, gay, bisexual, transsexual
MEHRC	Medical Ethics and Medical History Research Centre
MMC	Malaysian Medical Council
MoH	Ministry of Health
MOHME	Ministry of Health and Medical Education
MSM	Men who have sex with men
NBC	National Bioethics Committee
NCCR	National Committee for Clinical Research
OED	Oxford English Dictionary
OHRP	Office for Human Research Protections
OIC	Organisation of Islamic Cooperation
OXTREC	Oxford Tropical Research Ethics Committee

PMDC	Pakistan Medical and Dental Council
REC	Research ethics committee
SEA	South East Asia
TUMS	Tehran University of Medical Sciences
WHO	World Health Organization

1   Introduction

When you talk about values, for example, it's very difficult for people, for survivors of domestic violence, to actually just disconnect with their husband because they think that religion gives a certain interpretation about men and wives' relationships. Now, how do you tell a woman, a survivor, for example, about obedience? This is critical values when you talk about intimate kinds of violence in a Muslim culture … I realise this is not just Muslim culture, but in any faith community, in fact, because, in my studies, it comes up like 30% are Christians, 30% are Hindus and 30% are Muslim. They just come up naturally.

When you talk about obedience, for example, most of these religions, most of these believers of these religion, I'll put it that way, believe that women must obey their husbands, but they stop short there. When you want to engage them on this dialogue about what obedience is all about, you're really trying to intrude into their faiths, sometimes because you're trying to get them to have this dialogue with you. Sometimes, I wonder whether that is right to do, but, at the same time, I also wonder what would happen if you don't do. Will they just get stuck with that knowledge? Shouldn't we then engage them with this dialogue about the whole idea of obedience?

As a researcher, if you know you just don't want to engage them in this dialogue, then just leave them and go on with your research, continue to finish up your research. Who will then support them to continue with this dialogue, this religious dialogue that you have started with them? That is important, isn't it? Do we start this dialogue with them or not? If I don't do it, at the back of my mind, as a believer … I want to give them information, who can give this information? What kind of information … should [they] have so that they can process this whole idea about these rules that they have in mind about obedience so that they can be really knowledgeable, so that they can make the right decision?

As the quote above shows, ethical deliberations by researchers in practice reveals a complexity beyond an understanding and interpretation of international research ethics guidelines. The researcher explains the challenges she faces as a Public Health expert and social scientist seeking to enumerate and understand the prevalence of domestic and intimate partner violence within her own community. As a researcher she relies on guidelines to assist in outlining the aims and scope of her work, as well as the method. In practice, however, she encounters deep religious and cultural commitments of participants, which causes her to reflect on her own practice, motivations and moral concerns. Her experience reveals that guidelines are but one source of ethical deliberations for professionals working in contexts where their own religious and cultural commitments, as well as the faith of their participants, influence the types of research they undertake and how research is conducted.

For the researcher whose voice is captured in the quote, her work on intimate and domestic partner violence involves a complex nexus of moral resources including global ethics guidelines and training, a personal understanding of Islamic ethical values, cultural understandings of local norms as well as a shared responsibility and relationship to members of her community. Her reflections show that for Muslim researchers in such contexts, their moral universe is deeply informed by their own faith and the faith of their participants, where religious understandings inform their duty to participants as well as their professional role as researchers. The quote also highlights current limitations in our understandings of how bioethics is done in such contexts and that there is a scarcity of resources that researchers in such circumstances can rely on to help inform and support their work.

This volume is a modest attempt at addressing this knowledge gap by first providing an overview of the growing role of Islam within the biomedical research ethics discourse. This introductory chapter also outlines key Islamic ethico-legal theory pertinent for readers keen to know how Islam may inform bioethical discussions as well as providing an essential methodological backdrop for subsequent chapters. This is followed by a review of research guidelines published in Muslim contexts followed by an in-depth empirical study of research ethics in practice in two Muslim majority countries – Malaysia and Iran. The final chapter provides more extensive methodological detail for junior researchers and PhD candidates seeking to carry out similar research and analyses.

Why study the influence of Islam on biomedical research ethics?

Globally, Islam forms the second largest religious affiliation; yet reviewing the literature reveals that very little study has been done to explore its role in the context of research ethics (Suleman, 2016). This is pressing because there are 1.6 billion Muslims across the globe,[1] accounting for just under a quarter of the world's population. Pew Forum research further indicates that this number is rising exponentially. Additionally, the majority of Muslims live in the economic developing world and, therefore, can form a significant cohort for research as well as those who carry out the research. Normatively, Islam has generally encouraged the use of science, medicine and biotechnology as solutions to human suffering, and as such this study was

---

1 For more detailed population profile information on the world religions, please see Pew Research Center (2015, April 2). The future of world religions: Population growth projections, 2010–2050: Why Muslims are rising fastest and the unaffiliated are shrinking as a share of the world's population. https://assets.pewresearch.org/wp-content/uploads/sites/11/2015/03/PF_15.04.02_ProjectionsFullReport.pdf (Last accessed 15 January 2020).

designed to examine its influence, as a moral resource, on local ethical decision-making (Inhorn, 2008, pp. 252–6). Some authors have suggested that novel ethical dilemmas that have been presented by recent biomedical advancements in clinical medicine are functioning as a catalyst within the Islamic scholarly sphere, compelling religious experts into discussions about these challenges and the need for appropriate solutions (Sachedina, 2009, pp. 1–50). In relation to this claim, there is substantial literature on the influence of Islam within the clinical sphere and the need for religio-culturally competent care (Gatrad & Sheikh, 2001; Padela & Punekar, 2009; Inhorn & Serour, 2011; Ilkilic 2002). However, there has been no study on the impact of the Islamic tradition on research practice and how the role of the researcher/clinician is considered from this perspective.

In Muslim contexts, I was also keen to investigate the role religious views and values play in defining what counts as an ethical problem and what it means to be an ethical researcher. The latter is critical to gain a deeper understanding of the moral universe of Muslim researchers or the challenges researchers may face when working with a Muslim community. I also became keenly aware, through familiarisation with the Islamic bioethics literature and discussions with experts in the field, that within the Muslim tradition, although the formulation of religio-ethical opinions has customarily been perceived as the exclusive charge of religious scholars, more recently physicians and scientists themselves have taken on this task. One study has shown that Muslim medical and scientific experts are becoming involved in the drafting of Islamic legal rulings in an attempt to answer emerging religio-ethical challenges within the biomedical sphere (Ghaly, 2013a). Given such developments, I considered it pertinent to assess the nature of this emerging, multifaceted role of the Muslim physician/scientist/researcher and the impact it may have on the global health-research ethics discourse. Also, those who participate in research and their families may consider their Islamic faith important when making decisions about enrolling in trials. Such considerations may include issues relating to the Islamic conception of autonomy (Sachedina, 2009, p. 13); what the participants, families and broader public consider as the benefits and harms of research and which types of research questions and interventions are considered acceptable according to the Islamic faith. Very little study has been done to explore the influence of such factors on biomedical research ethics.

Studies have shown that between 2006–2010, there was a four percent rise in the number of drug trials conducted in the Middle East (Alahmad, et al., 2012), which accounts for a substantial portion of the world that ascribes to the Islamic faith. During that period, the Middle East accounted for the largest increase in such research compared to any other region in the world (Alahmad, et al., 2012). Muslim majority countries in South East Asia (SEA), such as Malaysia, Indonesia and Brunei, have also displayed a rise in biomedical research. However, some authors have suggested that one of the reasons for the outsourcing of clinical trials to countries in SEA is to avoid the rigorous governance mechanisms present in Europe and North American countries (Yusuf, 2014; Garrafa et al., 2010). Similarly, the Middle East has been considered a popular site for research due to improving infrastructure, patient diversity as well as fewer ethical constraints in comparison to Europe and North America (Alahmad, et al., 2012; Silverman, 2017). A study has shown that members of research ethics committees in Egypt considered the development of suitable national ethics guidelines a key priority (Sleem, et al., 2010). The establishment and evolution of research ethics guidelines and committees will be briefly discussed before returning to their development in the Muslim world[2] and their link to the Islamic faith.

Biomedical advancement and research ethics

Global wealth and development has been increasing rapidly, in a manner that is historically unprecedented. Despite this advancement, there is growing disparity in health measures, such as mortality, quality of life and disease incidence (Berlinguer, 2004). The global burden of disease is disproportionately large in developing countries, yet a fraction of medical research efforts are dedicated to the problems affecting the world's poorest people. Estimates have shown that less than ten percent of the world's medical research resources are employed for health problems in the developing world, where more than 90 percent of the disease burden lies ('the 10/90 gap') (Global Forum for Health Research, 2004). To address this disparity, the Ad Hoc Committee on Health Research (Lin, 1997) and the International Conference on Health Research for Development (COHERD)[3] have made five recommendations to stimulate more equitable distribution of medical research resources. These include: action to correct the 10/90 gap in research funding and to build the capacity of health research systems in developing countries; creation of international research networks and public-private partnerships; increased funding for health research by developing countries; and creation of health research forums to monitor progress (Global Forum for Health Research, 2004).

In recent years, biomedical research in developing countries has been expanding, with important implications for the development of novel, lifesaving therapies for pandemics such as HIV (Nuffield Council on Bioethics, 2002). It has also been suggested that health research conducted in developing countries may represent a valuable source of healthcare, a means of addressing conditions specifically affecting these areas, or a vehicle for implementing such solutions whilst capacity building in the form of infrastructure development and the training of local staff (Bhutta, 2002).

It is widely accepted that biomedical advancement has to be carefully monitored with sufficient governance processes to ensure there is no compromise on ethical standards (Lurie & Wolfe, 1997). Initially, lessons from the Nazi experiments (Weindling, 2008) and more recently Tuskegee (Curran, 1973) and Guatemala

2   The Muslim world in this study is defined as the countries that are members of the Organisation of Islamic Cooperation (OIC) (2020). http://www.oic-oci.org (Last accessed 15 January 2020).
3   Council on Health Research for Development (COHRED) (2000). International Conference on Health Research for Development, Bangkok. www.conference2000.ch (Last accessed 15 January 2020).

(Frieden & Collins, 2010) illustrated the importance of ethical oversight and high ethical standards to ensure participant safety and the protection of the local population's interests (Emanuel et al., 2004). Although trials on humans can be traced back several centuries, contemporary approaches to protect human subjects started only after the atrocities seen in Germany (Caballero, 2002). Following the Second World War, surviving Nazi doctors were prosecuted for war crimes at the Nuremberg Trials. The resulting military tribunal articulated the Nuremberg Code, in 1947 (Annas & Grodin, 2008). The code banned forced experiments in humans, setting the basis for the World Medical Association's Declaration of Helsinki a few years later in 1964. These landmark documents received general international support and led to the "universal" adoption of some key principles, such as the principle of independent, informed consent (Emanuel, et al., 2004). It is important to note, however, that there are those who have argued that the Nuremberg Code has had little effect on global research practices and that the code would only be applicable to totalitarian regimes (Caballero, 2002).

Recent work on global biomedical ethics has transformed dramatically, considering not only challenges in consent procedures (Freedman, 1987) but also more subtle questions relating to exploitation, the need for research to be responsive to local population needs and the sustainability of research. This shift has occurred, as there is growing realization that some of the most contentious contemporary ethical controversies are not related to informed consent but rather to the ethics of appropriate risk-benefit ratios, exploitation and the value of research to the local community (Emanuel, et al., 2000), where the endemic socioeconomic injustices also cannot be overlooked (IJsselmuiden, et al., 2010).

It is also important to note here that the field of global health research ethics faces the continuing challenge of its application within ethnographically diverse settings. Although bioethics has increasingly developed a global consciousness, some authors suggest that the universal principles to successfully guide ethical decision-making irrespective of cultural or religious contexts are not available and may never be established (Ryan, 2004; Chattopadhyay & De Vries, 2012). Despite the variety of work that has been accomplished thus far (in deriving ethical principles, applying them and reviewing them), there are concerns that many researchers fail to take into consideration the pertinence of religious pluralism, cultural differences and moral diversity, which pervades in different societies (Durante, 2008).

As mentioned above, the increase in clinical trials in the OIC countries emphasises the need for ensuring that these sites of clinical trials have a robust governance process, to ensure that the research that is taking place is ethical. The establishment of research ethics governance systems that can successfully oversee research and its development requires both intellectual and infrastructural investment. The latter will ensure that research being conducted within the OIC is ethically sound, avoids exploitation and produces results that are valid internationally. As a result, Muslim bioethicists in the region are now identifying factors relevant to clinical research within the top ten bioethical challenges facing Muslim countries, including: justice, human rights, bioethics capacity building and bioethics committees (Bagheri, 2014).

Furthermore, there have been claims that countries from within the Muslim world have developed "Islamic" guidelines (Kazim, 2007) for the ethical conduct of research. Yet there has been very little study of this "Islamic" influence on the ethical decision-making within the context of biomedical research in such settings. Chapter 2 provides a detailed analysis of said guidelines to review such claims. Another study has shown that three countries within the Middle East have drafted guidelines that "claim to respect Islamic law" (Alahmad, et al., 2012). Subsequent chapters evaluate what is defined as "Islamic law" and the latter's influence on biomedical research conduct.

Having discussed the importance of establishing research governance processes, the need for guidelines, and the challenge in establishing globally acceptable protocols, the next section briefly outlines the ongoing debates in bioethics on (i) normative versus empirical ethics; and (ii) whether the emphasis ought to be on the search for and application of universal values, or whether it ought to be accepted that what is more suitable are religio-culturally appropriate ethical principles and/or guidelines.

Normative versus empirical ethics

The relative contributions and validity of empirical and theoretical ethics in informing ethical norms has been discussed and debated since ancient times (Garrard & Wilkinson, 2005, pp. 77–92), and many authors now agree the vital role empirical ethics plays in informing normative ethics (Parker, 2012, pp. 131–52; Kon, 2009; Dunn, et al., 2012; Widdershoven, et al., 2008, pp. 1–68; Leget, et al., 2009). Those who argue against the employment of empirical methods in establishing ethical norms suggest there is a "gap" which exists between facts and values. This gap, they propose, prevents the derivation of ethical conclusions from empirical data (Kon, 2009).

There are two challenges that need to be made to such a claim. The first is that it is important to consider the impact of theoretical ethics on practice. In the context of research, it is not only important but a moral imperative to assess the extent to which our theoretical understanding of what ought to be done, which may be captured within guidelines, can provide the necessary foundation for ethical decision-making. If the purpose of the field of research ethics is to protect participants and support researchers' ability to make ethical decisions, then to ensure the improvement and sustainability of such a system requires some process of feedback into the theoretical framework. Just as clinical guidelines require input from clinical practice to ensure the guidelines are responsive to contextual changes (Garrard & Wilkinson, 2005, pp. 77–92), research ethics guidelines and infrastructures require the same governance processes to ensure they reflect theoretical ideals. Thus, if we wish to affect change in the research ethics discourse and practice, it is imperative we understand better the contextual application of the theory.

Secondly, we can use this empirical understanding to help refine our ethical norms. Kon (2009) described four ways in which empirical research can normatively inform clinical practice. Two of these are relevant to this discussion on research ethics. Empirical data, such as capturing the views of researchers and/or observing what they do, can inform normative ethics by contributing to an understanding of: (a) ideal versus reality and (b) the changing of ethical norms. This second factor is informed by empirical study and involves an ethical analysis of empirical findings, which may require multiple studies and publications to provide the necessary basis for a gradual shift in norms (Kon, 2009).

The aim of this research is to offer a distinctive account of the ways in which Islam and its associated practices are appropriated in the context of specific ethical issues within the field of biomedical research. The ethical analysis in this study will offer a rich empirical account of the roles that ethics plays in the lives and thinking of the participants, such as what is an ethical problem for them, and how they go about addressing it. This volume, therefore, straddles social science and bioethics research, by describing the moral universe of Muslim researchers or researchers working in the Islamic/Muslim context as a way of studying the influence of Islam in contexts where it may be considered an important source of ethico-legal guidance. Future work may add to this study and may develop the basis for refinement and/or shift in ethical norms. As the ensuing chapters will reveal, Islam does influence the ethical decision-making of researchers, REC (Research ethics committee) members and guideline developers. Given this empirical reality, a modest attempt will be made in Chapter 7 to consider what the implications of such findings should be on the broader global bioethics and Islamic bioethics discourse.

Universal ethics versus relativism and respect for religio-cultural diversity

There has been a long-standing debate within bioethics about whether ethical principles are dependent on time and space, and are therefore relative, or whether there are universally acceptable principles for determining ethical rightness and wrongness, even if the interpretation of these is highly dependent upon context. This modest volume will not offer an end to this debate; rather, it aims to add to the existing discussions by offering an understanding of how universal versus relativist considerations manifest in contexts where Islam is practiced as a faith and where Islam may be an important component of ethico-legal deliberations. The following brief summary presents of some of the arguments that will be relevant to analyses presented in subsequent chapters.

Those who consider the engagement with religio-cultural considerations a moral imperative argue that there exists a "Western" hegemony within bioethics (Chattopadhyay & De Vries, 2012). Ten Have argues that although many of the principles within bioethics have been formulated within "Western" countries, that need not imply that such values/principles are not valid outside of these contexts (ten Have, 2013). He suggests that religio-cultural considerations within bioethics as incorporated within the emerging field of Islamic bioethics "should not be understood as a separate bioethics; but it should be interpreted within the context of global bioethics" (ten Have, 2013, p. 614). I think it is important to highlight here that the emphasis within this book is not to suggest or stress a distinction between Islamic and global bioethics. Rather, it is to provide insight into how commonly accepted principles, such as autonomy, are understood and applied within Islamic/Muslim contexts and whether there are particular ethical and/or practical contextual challenges and/or considerations that are necessary when such principles are deliberated.

It is important to mention briefly that although now presented as secular, "Western" bioethics itself has its origins within religion and, more specifically, Christianity (Jonsen, 1998, pp. 34–59). Jonsen explores the birth of bioethics through prominent figures who originally trained in theology, but later their religious dominations and training faded to give way to the independent field of bioethics (Jonsen, 1998, pp. 34–59). In the Middle East and SEA, where the majority of Muslims reside, little is known about the influence of Islam in bioethics and, more particularly, research ethics, or how such an influence originated and is evolving. Again, the purpose of this volume is not to distinguish Islam from other religions or ethical influences. It is commonly understood that Islam shares many of the values and principles of other faiths, particularly Christianity and Judaism, with their shared Abrahamic roots. However, as very little is known about Islam's theological and legal influences on bioethical decision-making, it would be important to explore whether it plays a role in bioethical considerations in such contexts. If Islam does play a role, then it would be useful to explore how this influence manifests, who is involved, what tools are used to engage in bioethical questions and how such questions are defined and addressed. If during such an exploration there is evidence of distinctive ways of thinking about and addressing bioethical questions from the Islamic perspective, then these features will be emphasised.

Supporters of the idea that "bioethical principles (should) be derived from the moral traditions of local cultures" (Chattopadhyay & De Vries, 2012, p. 1) explain that universal principles to successfully guide ethical decision-making irrespective of cultural or religious contexts are not available and may never be established (Ryan, 2004; Chattopadhyay & De Vries, 2012). Furthermore, they suggest that insisting on and applying "universal" principles "does not promote respect and justice in medicine and medical research and can, in fact, cause real harm to persons" (Chattopadhyay & De Vries, 2012, p. 2) including an "irreparable loss of diversity" (Chattopadhyay & De Vries, 2012, p. 9).

Blum explains that within the existing literature there is very little consideration given to moral perception and particularity (Blum, 1994, pp. 30–44). He explains that although much is said about guidelines and rules, there is little deliberation about how a situation may "have a particular character for a particular moral agent" (Blum, 1994, pp. 30–44). Dancy explains that ethical narratives may not be narrowed into "a principle" per se, and what is considered a reason to act in one situation need not be considered the reason in another case (Dancy, 2004, pp. 1–12). Again, very little is known about such moral perceptions, particularity from the perspective of Muslim researchers, REC members, guideline developers and/or those who work with Muslim participants. This research is an attempt at considering such moral perceptions, particularity by exploring the moral universe of biomedical research stakeholders as a way of studying the influence of Islam in contexts where it may be considered an important source of ethico-legal guidance.

Others have explained that before principles/values can be considered universal, local people and traditions must be able to derive and articulate their own principles/values (Sachedina & Ainuddin, 2004, pp. 1–8) about what is commonly agreed and where the discordances lie. It is only then that a more balanced understanding can be achieved about whether such differences are simply related to non-moral facts, or if there are indeed distinctive values, frameworks and deliberative mechanisms characteristic of such local peoples and/or traditions.

In this book I will not be arguing about whether or not religion/culture ought to be involved in research ethics. Rather, the focus is on whether and how such an involvement occurs in the case of Islam and Muslims. The emphasis is on how, despite a global emphasis on universal norms, where Islam is predominately practiced and/or depended upon for ethico-legal decision-making, there is an inevitable influence of the Islamic faith, its ethico-legal tools and norms on aspects outside of traditional religious observance. How such an influence manifests within biomedical research ethics is poorly understood, and this research aims to address this knowledge gap. The aim is not to justify a role for religious/Islamic approaches to research ethics, rather it is to first explore how such an influence manifests and then to offer whether and how such influences can contribute to the broader global bioethical discourse.

The ethical reflections in this book focus on how concepts around research ethics and ethical guidelines are understood and implemented, and whether differing contexts present unique considerations that should inform our theoretical understanding of what ought to be done in the context of research. Some may argue that, despite contextual differences, ideals ought to be universal. So, even if we agree that some empirical work is necessary to inform our theoretical ideals, how far should this consideration go? Many of the ethical norms we have today are developed and empirically informed in the developed Western world. If, however, these ideals are needed and implemented for different contexts, then how far should we assume they are adequate in not only meeting the theoretical ideal but also whether the theoretical ideal we began with is ethically appropriate. Those who argue for moral universalism emphasize the shared human experience (ten Have, 2013; ten Have & Gordijn, 2010) and the dangers of moral relativism (Macklin, 1999, p. 24) providing a justification for atrocities, such those witnessed in Nazi Germany. The authors claim that moral relativism in the field of research ethics will lead to harm of already vulnerable research subjects (Bracanovic, 2010). There is also the argument that if we begin to consider each differing opinion, then it may be impossible to derive anything meaningful and consistent enough to ensure necessary ethical protections within research.

However, universalism presents its own challenges and dangers. If theoretical protections are formulated to serve the vulnerable and assist practitioners seeking to do the best that they can, then what happens if the theory challenges the pre-existing ideals of different communities? Such theoretical ideals, therefore, may harm the very communities they have been formulated to protect (Chattopadhyay & De Vries, 2012). Another important consideration is that religio-cultural experiences and phenomena inform theoretical norms and values (Shabana, 2013). Many authors have considered that "bioethics is an embedded socio-cultural practice" (Ives & Dunn, 2010, p. 256; Ives, et al., 2016), and so the theoretical considerations of ethicists of what ought to be done by practitioners cannot be detached from both the ethicists' and practitioners' personal and environmental contexts. Ives and Dunn (2010) propose that "moral intuitions" precede "moral arguments", and "our intuitions can be shaped over time by our life experiences" (Ives & Dunn, 2010, p. 259). They go on to explain that "moral argument is almost always a rationalisation, explanation or justification of a moral intuition linked to an instinct that is distinctly personal" (Ives & Dunn, 2010, p. 259).

This research is, therefore, a starting point for understanding if and how Islam influences biomedical research ethics. Although international guidelines have been adapted to incorporate Islamic views, studies have shown that the latter are of limited practical application within a "Muslim country" setting (Sleem, et al., 2010). As yet it is unclear whether Muslim researchers rely on such adapted guidelines or simply use the existing international guidelines that are present. If the latter is true, then it may be useful to assess how Muslim researchers employ "secular" guidelines within their local environment and whether they need to adapt them based on their faith and/or context.

In settings where non-Muslim researchers are working with a majority Muslim population, it may be valuable to assess whether they are able to apply research protocols according to international guidelines, verbatim, or whether adaptation is necessary based on local religious beliefs. For example, recruitment of women may have to be done with the consent of husbands or male relatives. Also, it would be valuable to assess the practical ethics struggles faced by Muslim researchers/physicians, for example, ensuring that research is conducted in compliance with the *Shariah* (Islamic law). The latter may be comprised of a mixture of secular and religious thinking and principles. Both of these aspects of study will enable greater understanding of how Islam influences the expectations and experience of research participants and the dilemmas and decisions of Muslim and non-Muslim researchers when working in Islamic/Muslim contexts.

It is important to emphasise here that the relationship between a particular population or sub-group, its religious practices and the broader historical and cultural situation is complex and can be context specific. In turn, these context-specific complexities may well influence the relationship between both the Islamic texts and the ethical issues with which they are confronted within research. The aim of this study is not to simplify or reduce such complexities; rather, it is an attempt at characterising some of the resulting tensions that arise at the interface of these different factors. The relationship between Islamic texts, scholarship, interpretation and the lived practice of Islam is a complex and evolving one, and this volume is a step towards evaluating how such factors influence the understanding of ethics issues in research.

Although I have used religion and culture interchangeably so far, and many have argued that religion and culture are different even if inextricably linked (Sachedina, 2009, pp. 14–9), it is important to briefly explore how the terms religion and culture will be used in this volume and, more specifically, in relation to Islam and its cultures.

Religion and culture – commonalities, incongruities and challenges

Culture is an equivocal concept, often meaning different things to different people. Therefore, it is important to consider carefully how it will be referred to in this book, and how culture relates to religion. Some anthropologists have defined culture as a "total way of life of a discrete society, its traditions, habits, beliefs and art" which has "certain constant features … that differentiate it from other cultures in other times or places" (Clausen, 1996, p. 380). Others have suggested that it is "an organised way of life which is based on a common tradition and conditioned by a common environment" (Dawson, 2013, p. 35). Dawson explains, therefore, that "a common way of life involves common standards of value and consequently a culture is a spiritual community which owes its unity to common beliefs" (Dawson, 2013, p. 36). Although the definitions of such scholars help to delineate culture and identify its relation with religion, there are limitations to the application of such definitions in reference to Islam and its many cultures.

Islam is a religion with a set of beliefs, values, traditions and normative texts. However, Islam, as with any other religion, cannot exist without being interpreted and lived within a culture (Ramadan, 2009, p. 183). Since its inception, Islam has spread as a faith system to many different cultures across the globe. As a religion, therefore, it has been interpreted and lived through many different cultures. These cultures include the original culture of the Prophet Muhammad's community in Arabia, the evolution of that Arabian culture and the cultures within which Islam spread globally from China to Spain. Such interpretation and application of the normative texts continues to this day where Muslims may reside as a minority or majority community across the globe. It may be suggested that the constant features of the religion and its practices can be identified and therefore distinguished from these cultures. Marshall Hodgson has offered the valuable term, "Islamicate", which helps to distinguish elements found within Muslim societies that are outside of Islam, yet intrinsically linked to Muslim culture. This so-called Islamicate "would refer not directly to the religion, Islam, itself, but to the social and cultural complex historically associated with Islam and the Muslims, both among Muslims themselves and even when found among non-Muslims" (Hodgson, 1977a, p. 59). The term Islamicate, therefore, helpfully enables us to refer to the cultural elements expressed by Muslims considered outside of Islam.

However, Islam has within it the accepted tradition of textual interpretation that is dependent on these evolving cultures. Padela (2013) explains that within the Islamic ethico-legal discourse, when the normative texts are silent, local custom (*urf*) can be used to inform the law and is considered a secondary source within the Islamic ethico-legal framework. Such customs or cultural elements are therefore not simply part of an Islamicate; rather, they contribute to what is considered "Islamic" or the religion proper. The context or culture is not only a source of textual interpretation, but also the space within which religious norms and laws are practiced and where an understanding of values is developed.

Why is it important to make a distinction between Islam and its cultures? It is essential to be able to confidently identify a practice, value or belief as "Islamic" versus one that is outside of the faith, but simply assumed as being "Islamic" by someone who is Muslim. This is because Islam as a religious entity has the ability to afford religious authority to cultural beliefs and practices. Customs that are used to interpret religious texts can be labelled as norms within Islamic law. Therefore, it may serve the interests of some to classify their values as "Islamic" rather than these simply being intrinsic to their culture or personal preference. Tariq Ramadan (2009) explains that the universality of Islam's message is in its integration of "cultural specificities so long as they do not contradict [the] religion's formal injunctions" and "in allowing for [the] critical assessment of the surrounding cultural reference" (p. 188). The latter is an essential feature of Islam, where as a belief system it not only takes from the cultures within which it resides, but also impresses upon these cultures a nurturing towards its higher values of peace, reconciliation and justice.

Bioethical decision-making is dependent on a personal and/or collective consideration of values, which, as explained above, may be considered universal or contextual. Within this volume, there is a focus on these contextual norms that reside within Islamic/Muslim communities and the identification of issues where the distinction between culture and religion is pertinent.

Having briefly explained why studying the influence of Islam on research ethics would be a valuable endeavour and having provided some background to the debates around universal and relative considerations in ethics and the complexities around Islam and its cultures, I will present an overview of Islam, its origins, history and ethico-legal tradition. This background is the basis upon which subsequent chapters are developed.

Islam: Its origins

Over 1,400 years ago, in the Arabian dessert, a man named Muhammad spoke to his people of having received revelation from God. Muhammad at the time was illiterate, and the message he conveyed, profound. His family and friends who knew him as an honest man were equal in accepting and rejecting his faith. Yet, the religion he preached grew in enormous popularity in the Arabian Peninsula within just a few years. During his lifetime Muhammad formed a community that excelled in moral, socio-political and economic pursuits (Lings, 2012, pp. 332–4). At the time of the Prophet's death in 632 AD, he had successfully united the numerous tribes of Arabia into a powerful nation. The latter extended from the Atlantic Ocean in the West, to the borders of China in the East (Syed, 1981). The Arabs did not destroy, but rather assimilated the cultures and knowledge of the people they ruled.

Muhammad taught his followers, like his predecessor Abraham, the Glory and Oneness of God. Muslims consider the book/revelation he received, the *Qur'an*, and his tradition (compiled in books of *Hadith*) not simply as a collection of religious rituals, but a "complete way of life" (Winter & Williams, 2003, p. 3). Thus, Muslims rely on the scriptural sources (the *Qur'an* and *Hadith*) as their moral compass for all facets of life – private and public. The consideration of the sources of moral guidance is critical in Islam, as in any other faith. The normative sources and development of Islamic ethics will now be briefly discussed.

Islamic ethics: Normative sources and development

Ethics is concerned with determining the rightness and wrongness of actions, decisions or goals (Singer, 1994, pp. 3–10). There has been growing interest in ethics in professional spheres, such as medicine, as a result of historical atrocities, as explained above. Pertaining to ethics, Islam places a great emphasis on moral virtues. The comparable word for ethics in Islam is a combination of two words, *aqhlaq*, meaning proper conduct, and *adab*, or virtue (Siddiqui, 1997). Muhammad lived his life as an example of virtue, mild temperament and exceptional character. He stated that he "was sent to perfect good character" (Mālik, Book 47, Number 47.1.8). When his companions asked: "'O Messenger of God, what is the best thing that a person may be given?' He said: 'Good manners'" (Ibn Majah, Book 31, Hadith 3436) or *aqhlaq*. There have been numerous works on the "science of virtues" (*ilm al-aqhlaq*) and vast amounts of literature on *adab* (Sartell & Padela, 2015).

During the expansion of the Islamic civilisation and the translation of Greek texts into Arabic, Greek virtue ethics were incorporated into the Islamic civilisation by scholars such as al-Kindi, al-Farabi and Miskawayh (Fakhry, 2009, pp. 1–77). However, very little is known about the influence of such sciences and their evolution on the moral decision-making of contemporary Muslim societies, physicians and biomedical researchers. This research examines the values/virtues from within the Islamic tradition that guide Muslim researchers and how such values/virtues are encountered, upheld, implemented or reconciled within the field of biomedical research.

Authors such as Fakhry argue that the *Qur'an*, upon which the Muslim moral and social life revolves, does not contain ethical theories per se, though it "embodies the whole of the Islamic ethos" (Fakhry, 1991, p. 1). He explains, however, that a student of Islamic ethics may elicit this ethos by referring to sources that are rooted in the *Qur'an* (Fakhry, 1991, pp. 1–10). These include Quranic exegesis (*tafsir*), jurisprudence (*fiqh*) and scholastic theology (*kalam*). Contemporary Muslim scholars thus rely on a combination of these and the primary sources (*Qur'an* and *Hadith*) to derive guidance and rulings when tasked with ethical problems.

It is important to highlight here that the primary sources of Islam, namely the *Qur'an* and *Hadith*, require interpretation for distinguishing between right and wrong. Many authors describe moral reasoning for Muslims as being comprised of a combination of one's intuitive nature (*fitr'a*), reason (*aql*) and revelation (*wahy*) (Al-Bar & Chamsi-Pasha, 2015, pp. 4–5). The balance of these sources of moral reasoning must be explored briefly within Islam's history, as the theological difference between the sects that emerged within Islam differ in their reliance on intuition, reason and revelation. The differences seen within Islam's schools of theology (*kalam*) echo the differences observed amongst scholars of other religions, including Judaism and Christianity (Adamson, 2015, pp. 30–46). Also, within Islam, the normative texts do not directly outline the objectives or values of the Islamic law (*Shariah*). These objectives have to be derived from the source texts and then applied to emerging questions/problems. The formation of two key schools of theology and the development of the objectives of the *Shariah* will be briefly discussed now. These elements of Islamic ethics will be relevant in later chapters as they help to explain the underlying reasoning behind certain ethico-legal decisions within Islamic/Muslim contexts.

Sources of morality: Reason and revelation in Islam and the formation of the Ash'ari and Mu'tazili schools of theology – drawing key distinctions between the Sunni and Shi'i schools of law

One of the most important features of Islam's history is the establishment of the *Sunni* and *Shi'i* schools of law. Following the Prophet Muhammad's death, tensions arose about who should succeed him as the Commander of the Believers. Followers of Islam are considered to be in two main branches. Those who accepted Abu Bakr, Muhammad's closest friend and confidante, as his successor are known as *Sunnis* (followers of communal tradition) – who are divided into four recognised schools of law. Others who instead paid allegiance to Ali, Muhammad's nephew and son in law, came to be known as *Shia* (partisans of Ali). Muslims are divided into 80 percent *Sunnis* and 20 percent *Shia*. The division is not only political, but also religious. *Sunnis*, after the Prophet's death, placed their authority in the *Sunnah* (Prophetic tradition) and the community (*jama'a*). The *Shias*, in contrast, placed authority not only in the Prophet but also in the descendants of Ali, or the infallible imam. *Shi'i* philosophy and theology is heavily influenced by *Mu'tazili* theology, which emphasised free will and the role of reason in the interpretation of the *Qur'an* and *Hadith* (Winter, 2008, pp. 1–14). Tremayne (2009) reports that *Shi'i* scholars' reliance on reason (*ijtihad*) to interpret the *Qur'an*, a practice she describes as "unique to the *Shia* sect" (p. 147), has led to the development of a more fluid religious interpretation within the *Shi'i* legal system, in comparison to the *Sunni* system (pp. 144–63). Furthermore, the *Ash'ari* school of theology, which was predominately inherited by the *Sunnis*, defined "good" and "bad" based primarily upon revelation, and they suggested that rationality be used when there is no text. Thus, the *Mu'tazili*'s answer to Plato's Euthyphro dilemma (Plato, 1914) would be that good and evil can be determined by the intellect. Whereas the *Ash'aris* would argue that good and evil can only be determined by God. This theological or "deistic subjectivism" (Padela, 2013) is a feature of the *Sunni* school.

As the *Sunni* school considers good as being determined by God's command, then these commands are known through revelation. Revelation has been circumscribed by the *Qur'an* and *Hadith*. Yet, both of these sources of revelation, as explained above, require contextual interpretation. Such interpretation depends on reason. Within the *Sunni* school, two secondary tools of legal reasoning are employed, namely *Ijma* (consensus of scholars) and *Qiyas* (analogical reasoning). The *Shi'i* school relies not on *Qiyas* but *ijtihad* or independent scholarly reasoning. Again, the relevance of this plurality in moral reasoning and the resulting differences will be explored in subsequent chapters.

Thus, reason and revelation find themselves inextricably linked within both the *Ash'ari* and *Mu'tazili* schools of theology and also in the subsequent *Sunni* and *Shi'i* schools of law. The weighting of reason and revelation, however, does differ in the different schools. In both schools, however, the authority to interpret scripture and derive laws is key, and the challenges that arise within contemporary Islam, in terms of "speaking in God's name" (El Fadl, 2014), will be explored in later chapters.

This theological and ethico-legal departure between the *Sunni* and *Shi'i* schools is pertinent for understanding and delineating some of the analyses made in Chapters 3 through 6. It is important to highlight here that contemporary *Sunni* and *Shi'i* scholars apply differing approaches to emerging bioethical questions. Often their conclusions differ starkly, not just because of the theological (*Ash'ari* and *Mu'tazili*) differences, but also due to complex ethico-legal, historic and sociological factors (Inhorn, 2012).[4] Some of the ethico-legal nuances between the two traditions will be examined in more detail in Chapters 3 and 4.

The higher objectives of the Shariah *(Islamic Law)* – Maqasid al Shariah

Within the *Sunni* school there has been a long-standing discussion about how the Islamic normative sources do not directly indicate the values or objectives of the *Shariah* (Islamic law derived from the normative texts). Centuries of scholarship have been dedicated to discerning these underlying values and principles of the *Shariah*. The school of *Maqasid* (higher objectives of the *Shariah*) questions what these underlying values may be. The search for the higher objectives of the *Shariah* began 1,000 years ago with scholars such as al-Juwayni (d. 1185), his student Abul Hamed al-Ghazali (d. 1111), al-Shatibi (d. 1388) and, more recently, Ahmed ar-Raysuni. They emphasise five key objectives: Preservation of (1) Faith, (2) Life, (3) Intellect, (4) Progeny, and (5) Property (Ramadan, 2009, pp. 59–76). Al Shatibi, in his pioneering work *al-Muwafaqat*, translated by ar-Raysuni (Raysuni, 2005, pp. 264–82), highlights the importance remaining faithful to the Divine intent by ensuring the understanding and application of the *Maqasid* in light of the conditions and needs of

---

4 For a more extensive background on different Islamic bioethics approaches between *Sunni* and *Shi'i* scholars, please see Marcia Inhorn's insightful ethnographic work on reproductive technologies (Inhorn, M. C. (2012). *Local babies, global science: Gender, religion and in vitro fertilization in Egypt*. Routledge).

the context. Other scholars have built on this idea and have suggested an expansion on the five objectives to also include the broader instructions or emphasis of the *Shariah* on justice and compassion.[5] Very little is known about how the application and reconciliation of the *Maqasid* works within the practice of biomedical research. Chapters 4 and 5 will provide a detailed empirical account of deliberations involving the *Maqasid* in practice.

Islamic bioethics and the role of fiqh

Islamic bioethics finds its roots in the same sources mentioned above. Since Islam's inception, Muslim physicians have paid special attention to ethics in their personal and professional practice (Zahedi, et al., 2009). Scholars within the Islamic tradition have always been aware of the moral underpinnings of the religious duties that all Muslims are required to fulfil. They validate their research upon the Islamic sources, when faced with practical questions, by ensuring they consider the many moral facets of each case (Sachedina, 2009, p. 7). Legal decisions, within Islamic jurisprudence (*fiqh*), are made after ensuring that meticulous attention is paid to the various factors that determine the rightness and wrongness of the matter under consideration. *Fiqh* is thus a robust juridical system rooted in the primary sources, analysed and applied by scholars to arrive at solutions to practical problems faced by Muslims. So Islamic bioethics can be considered a combination of virtue ethics, which focuses on the conduct of the practitioner (Al-Bar & Chamsi-Pasha, 2015, pp. 75–84), and legal ethics, which concerns the ethico-legal deliberation by scholars (*fiqh*) and the tradition upon which they rely. This tradition or the *Shariah*, which is often translated as "Islamic law", is more accurately understood as "a way or a well-trodden path to water" (Al-Bar & Chamsi-Pasha, 2015, pp. 6–7).

The deliberative tools employed within Islamic bioethics discourses include *fatawah* (singular *fatwah*) or non-binding ethico-legal Islamic opinions issued by a qualified Islamic jurists (known as a *mufti* or *faqih*) through individual reasoning (*ijtihad*) or by a *majma* or collective body of scholars who deliberate on emerging issues to arrive at collective *ijtihad*. In recent decades we have seen the institutionalization of collective *ijtihad*, through collaborations between legal schools and ministries of health (for example, the Islamic Juridical Council of the World Muslim League in Mecca, Saudi Arabia). Such bodies have been responsible for regularly reviewing and responding to emerging bioethical questions.[6]

---

5   When Umar (Commander of the Believers) stopped the cutting of the hands during the famine – he showed how the objective of justice overruled the text. Please see: Ramadan, T. (2009). *Radical reform: Islamic ethics and liberation*. New York: Oxford University Press.

6   For more background on sources of Islamic bioethics and Islamic normative sources, please see: Sachedina, A. A. (2009). *Islamic biomedical ethics: Principles and application*. New York: Oxford University Press. For a more detailed account on *Shariah*, see: Hallaq, W. B. (2009). *Shari'a: Theory, practice, transformations*. Cambridge: Cambridge University Press.

Furthermore, Muslim jurists have successfully derived legal and moral principles that evolved from their rulings. Sachedina (2009) refers to a few of these principles within his seminal work on Islamic Biomedical Ethics. Some of these principles, such as *Maslaha* (public good), *Dharurah* (necessity) and *Urf* (custom), will be explored in more detail in subsequent chapters. Little study has been done to explore how such principles are applied within the context of biomedical research ethics in Islamic/Muslim contexts. Having briefly outlined a history of Islam, its normative sources and the foundations of Islamic ethics and bioethics, I will now summarize the focus and methods of this study.

How can the empirical study of Muslim beliefs and practices inform an understanding of normative Islam?

One of the objectives of this research is to investigate whether and how people's personal religious beliefs impact their understanding and approaches to biomedical research ethics. If we accept the relevance of empirical study in informing ethical norms and the significance of religio-cultural input in deciding what is ethically appropriate in a given context, then how can the study of believers of a particular faith add to our normative understanding of that faith?

Within the literature, there resides a dichotomy. Some authors argue that no cohesive or "monolithic Islam" exists on medical matters (Brockopp & Eich, 2008). Whereas others consider the normative texts of Islam and what is derived from them as being unifying. Those who argue against a "monolithic Islam" consider the ethical encounters of Muslims within the medical sphere that are subsequently addressed by scholars as a compilation of Muslim medical ethics (Brockopp & Eich, 2008). As Islam has multiple branches, and the followers often consider each subsection an independent entity, the authors argue it may not be possible to arrive at a unified series of principles pertaining to medical matters rooted in one Islam. Thus, they do not consider the study of people of faith as a means of generating normativity about that faith (Brockopp & Eich, 2008, pp. 1–15).

However, despite there being contextual differences, rulings that are derived by Islamic scholars and applied by Muslims, although adapted to their local setting, are rooted in the *Qur'an*, the *Hadith* and/or the derived sciences. As a believing community, Muslims live their lives and arrive at decisions on how to conduct themselves ensuring that they are in accordance with God's will, as instructed in the *Qur'an* and *Hadith* and through consultation with scholars and/or pre-existing scholarly rulings. The latter sources that undergird the rulings are unanimously accepted as "Islamic". Of course it is important to highlight here that resources from within the Islamic tradition may be one of many different sources that Muslim researchers rely on for their ethical deliberations. It is, therefore, important to consider how best to determine what aspects of their decision-making rely specifically on "Islamic" sources. Direct questioning regarding underlying reasons and motivations may help with this distinction. Thus, by observation and direct questioning, Muslim laity may provide an understanding of how Islam is embodied. So, by studying Muslim behaviour, practices and views, and the use of scripture, law and scholarly edicts in the context of specific ethical issues, we can derive an understanding of normative Islam and its influence on biomedical research ethics.

Figure 1.1, which summarises the hierarchy of the sources of ethics and law in Islam, highlights where Muslim laity lies in the hierarchy and illustrates that the two primary sources of Islam are the *Qur'an* and *Hadith*. These sources have been interpreted, using legal tools such as *Ijma, Qiyas* and *Ijtihad*, to derive secondary sciences such as *fiqh*. In this study, therefore, I consider the normative sources of Islam to be the textual sources (*Qur'an* – word of God revealed to the Prophet Muhammad, and Hadith – traditions of the Prophet), the derived sciences: jurisprudence (*fiqh*), theology, *tasawwuf* (*Sufism*), *Adab* and *Aqhlaq*. Finally, the third level is that of the practice of Muslims as an embodiment of the textual sources and derived sciences. Although there is plurality within Islam, the source texts (*Qur'an* and *Hadith*) and sciences (*fiqh*, theology and *taswwuf*) carry an authoritative weight as well as an instructive component that is enacted through the behaviour of Muslims. Each of these elements, therefore, contributes to what is understood as the normative sources of Islam (Padela, 2013). These elements are foundational in understanding what participants in this study considered "what ought to be done" from an Islamic perspective. These recognised "Islamic" normative sources need to be distinguished from other sources of normativity, such as culture, that may also influence participants' decisions on "what ought to be done". As explained above, this distinction may be important in terms of delineating the normative

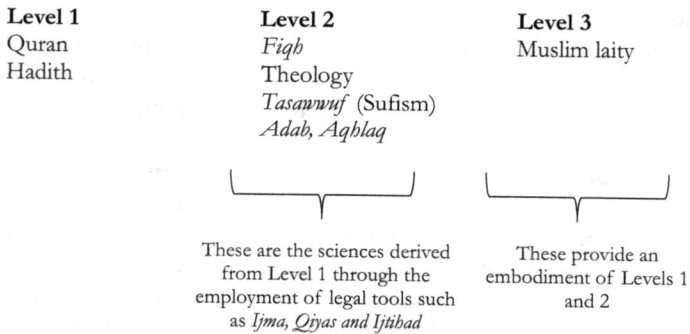

Level 1	Level 2	Level 3
Quran	*Fiqh*	Muslim laity
Hadith	Theology	
	Tasawwuf (Sufism)	
	Adab, Aqhlaq	

These are the sciences derived from Level 1 through the employment of legal tools such as *Ijma, Qiyas* and *Ijtihad*	These provide an embodiment of Levels 1 and 2

Figure 1.1 **The three levels of the normative sources of Islam and how the different levels interrelate**[7]

7   This schematic is adapted from: Ramadan, T. (2019). *Islamic ethics: A very short introduction.* Oxford: Oxford University Press. The pre-print manuscript was made available to attendees of a March 2016 two-day conference organised by the Jibreel Institute in collaboration with CILE (Research Center for Islamic Legislation and Ethics).

influence of Islam and its sources from other sources of normativity, such as the cultures of Muslims, in order to better understand the factors that influence decision-making in the biomedical research context.

The focus of the research findings presented in subsequent chapters is on the study of Muslims and how they understand and employ the sources in levels 1 and 2. This study is, therefore, a social science study of how Muslims respond to specific ethical challenges, with "Islam" (defined by the textual sources and derived sciences – levels 1 and 2) as one input (Padela, 2013). A study of Muslims can provide insight into the lived reality of what it means to embody Islam (Padela, 2013) – it can provide an understanding of the questions that Muslims face and how these are addressed. The practice of Muslim researchers and participants can provide a window into how Islam influences biomedical research.

Another reason for empirically studying the understanding and practice of Muslim researchers is that they may express certain beliefs, reasons or values that are simply cultural, not rooted in but supported by religious scripture. It would be important to empirically study what the role of religion is in such contexts and what practices are legitimized through the appropriation of religious texts. One of the objectives of this study is to investigate the influence of local cultures and traditions on how Islam influences ethical decision-making in the research context. An empirical study is suitable for challenging participants' views and gaining a better understanding of the underlying values and reasons for their ethical decision-making.

An additional consideration is that my review of the ethics guidelines (Chapter 2) and the literature (Suleman, 2016) showed that there is little from Islam's scriptural sources, scholarly texts and deliberations that relates directly to biomedical research ethics. Does this mean that Islam does not influence the work of Muslim researchers or research ethics committee members or that the tradition is not a necessary and/ or suitable resource when defining or dealing with bioethical problems in the research context? Or is there empirical evidence for the influence of Islam on biomedical research ethics that needs to be better understood?

Is it possible to study the influence of Islam and the role of Muslim contexts within the research ethics sphere without empirical methods? It may be possible to do a hypothetical study of how faith may influence the ethical decision-making of researchers or the types of questions that may arise when working with a faith based community; however, the aim of this study is to try and ascertain distinct moral problems that arise within the context of Islam and how these are addressed. The latter aim makes an empirical approach more suitable. An additional important consideration is that, within Islamic jurisprudence, the numerous schools of thought, although rooted in the same primary sources, may arrive at differing and often contradictory judgements (Kyriakides-Yeldham, 2005). It makes it all the more important, therefore, to study the lived reality of Muslim researchers to understand better whether and how they consult such sources and the impact of these on their ethical decision-making.

The guideline search and review has highlighted that consultation with researchers, Islamic scholars and physicians is key in order to understand the process by which ethical questions pertaining to research are chosen, prioritised and addressed through a process of communal enquiry. Little work has been done to understand in more detail the dynamics of meetings comprising of scholars of religious texts and the biomedical research context. It was considered pertinent, therefore, to capture the views, experiences and the challenges faced by the individuals involved in these processes to better understand how Islam influences biomedical research ethics.

What will be the empirical approach in this research?

Having explored the above theoretical considerations, it is important to outline that different empirical approaches may lead to distinctive conclusions being drawn. For example, it is important to reflect on what can be said generally about Islam and the thinking and practice of Muslims in the context of biomedical research. It is also important to consider how the investigation of the influence of Islam on biomedical research ethics can have implications for the broader discourse on Islamic bioethics and bioethics more generally.

There are two possible approaches to investigating the ways in which the practice of Islam and the interpretation and application Islamic texts and sciences are taken to feature in the understanding of ethics issues in research. The first would be to focus on exploring the complexities of the relationship between religious texts, religious practices and ethics in the context of specific ethical issues, such as genome research and tissue storage, as identified in the guideline (Chapter 2) and literature review (Suleman, 2016). The advantage of this approach would be that the specific ethical issues would frame the discussion of the other larger issues, such as the role of culture and Islamic scholars. However, the disadvantage would be that such an approach may not enable an understanding of ethical issues that may exist outside of the remit of those specified. The second method would be to concentrate on a particular set of contexts or communities and, in such a context, explore a wider range of issues. The advantage would be that such an open approach might yield an array of issues that would otherwise be missed by the first approach. The disadvantage would be that the claims about Islam and religious practices would be less generalisable.

Having considered both options, in order to optimise both breadth and depth of study, I decided to use a combination of these methods. The interviews were conducted in Malaysia and Iran using an amalgamation of prescribed questions or scenarios relating to research ethics issues identified in the literature and guideline review (e.g., tissue storage), as well as more open-ended questions to enable participants to share their views and experiences of other challenges and questions they face in their work. The feasibility of implementing a combination of these approaches has been central when making selections of study sites, drafting of topic guides and interview questions and selection of research participants (further details of which can be found in Chapter 8).

Research question and objectives

Against this background, the aim of this research was to assess if and how Islam influences ethical decision-making of researchers, REC members, guideline developers and Islamic scholars in the biomedical research context.

The specific objectives of the research are:

1   To investigate whether and how the institutional aspects of Islam, the normative texts, scholarship and the subsequent interpretation and derived sciences influence the understanding of ethical issues in biomedical research;
2   To study the emerging, multifaceted role of the Muslim researcher as a biomedical expert, and one who is keen to adopt the language of Islamic theology and law to define and address bioethical questions in the research context;
3   To investigate whether and how Islam responds to global health challenges, such as the ethical issues emerging from HIV/AIDS;
4   To study the influence of local cultures and traditions on how Islam influences ethical decision-making in the research context;
5   To investigate whether and how researchers' personal religious beliefs impact their understanding and approaches to biomedical research ethics; and
6   To study the intellectual deliberations of participants through an ethical analysis of the participants' understanding of normative ethical principles, and to develop my own account of what ethical challenges exist and/or arise within research contexts with Muslim researchers and/or Muslim participants.

Conclusion and chapter outlines

Islam, its texts and lived practice, finds growing importance within the global discourse on bioethics, as there is an increasing Muslim population and burgeoning interest in biomedical research and biotechnologies in the Muslim world. The aim of this book is to present the findings of primary research evaluating research ethics guidelines as well as an empirical qualitative study of stakeholder perceptions and ethical analysis. The book provides unique insight into how Islam and the moral commitments of Muslims influence the ethical decision-making of researchers, REC members, guideline developers and Islamic scholars in the biomedical research context.

This chapter provided a background to the research and introduced the need to understand better whether and how Islam influences biomedical research ethics. It briefly presented a history of Islam, its normative sources and an outline of the theory underlying Islamic ethics that will be relevant for subsequent chapters. It presented the research question and articulated six distinct but interrelated research objectives. The rest of this volume is organised into seven distinct but related chapters.

Chapter 2 reviews and explores the biomedical research ethics guidelines at the international, regional, national, state and institutional levels, which are employed within countries with a significant Muslim population. The review investigates the role of Islam, its normative sources and the Muslim context in such guidelines. The method of the review will also be presented here. The guideline and literature review (Suleman, 2016) were carried out to provide a broad overview of the knowledge and themes within biomedical research ethics pertaining to Islam and Muslims. As an understudied area, the themes presented an important guide for the empirical study and the remainder of this research. The guideline review also highlighted which countries have research ethics guidelines, providing a short list of potential sites for the empirical study.

An empirical study was carried out in two case study sites (2014–2015) to assess the extent to which Islam influences ethical decision-making within the context of biomedical research. 56 semi-structured interviews were carried out in Malaysia (38) and Iran (18) with researchers, REC members, guideline developers and Islamic scholars to understand whether Islam influences what they consider to be an ethico-legal problem, and if the latter emerges, then how such issues are addressed.

Having analysed the literature and guidelines, completed the interviews and studied the transcripts using a framework analysis, I identified four key topics that helped me organise my thoughts about the data and the insights emerging from the data. These four topics are the focus of the data chapters (Chapters 3 through 6). The following is a synopsis of these chapters:

Chapter 3 – The first topic is how Islam influences the understanding of ethics in research, through its institutional forms (religious texts, scholars and their legal edicts) that are encountered within particular structures, policies and laws nationally. This chapter also explains that, although these institutional forms of Islam broadly provide a permissive and flexible method of practical deliberation through *ijtihad* in deriving *fatawah*, there are emerging constraints and complexities in relation to what has traditionally been recognised as the Islamic scholarly authority. Although the task of *ijtihad* and issuing *fatawah* has been seen traditionally as the role of Islamic scholars, one of the striking features of the data analysis is that there is increasing involvement from biomedical experts (contextual scholars who are also informally trained in the Islamic sciences) and "bridge-scholars" (those formally being trained in biomedicine and the Islamic sciences) in this practical reasoning process.

Chapter 4 – The second topic is how the latter institutional forms of Islam, within the case study sites, face challenges from social and global changes. This chapter will present the Islamic responses to ethical issues in HIV/AIDS research. The ethical issues arising from HIV/AIDS require Islamic responses, as the epidemic raises issues about behavioural practices that are illegal in Islam, such as intravenous drug use, homosexuality and prostitution. This chapter presents a more substantive account of the ethical issues emerging from HIV/AIDS research and the use of *ijtihad* to derive *fatawah* as a unique mechanism of practical deliberation in Islam.

Chapter 5 – The third topic that was identified in my analysis is how the question of women's autonomy raises ethical challenges for researchers. At the level of researchers and RECs, the data show that there is a variation in understanding of what ought to be done when enrolling women in research, and particular challenges emerge when trying to conduct studies involving intimate/domestic partner violence and the sexual health and sexual experience of women.

Chapter 6 – The fourth topic that will be discussed is that the individuals within the institutional forms of Islam, such as biomedical researchers, REC members, guideline developers, and scholars, are personally struggling with balancing different priorities and value systems, including their own faith. When faced with a practical problem, such as the need to address the HIV/AIDS epidemic or whether and how to enrol women into a research study, the data show that researchers in these contexts concurrently have to consider what is recommended by physicians' codes of conduct, research ethics guidelines, global health priorities, as well as what is instructed by Islam and its formal structures together with local cultural values. The analysis suggests that researchers in such contexts, who are required to adopt multiple roles and balance numerous value systems and priorities, may face moral anxiety and frustration. Also, in addressing such practical challenges, respondents express a deep commitment to Islamic ethics and law, which influences their understanding of their legal and moral accountability.

Chapter 7 – The chapter discusses the findings presented in Chapters 3 through 6. It aims to synthesize and reflect further on the themes presented in the preceding chapters. It also presents an overview of the study and the ramifications for the broader field of biomedical research ethics, Islamic bioethics and future research. This chapter brings the findings to a close by presenting an overview of the key conclusions, emerging questions and tentative suggestions for future research for an area of study that is in its gestation.

In summary, the empirical study indicates five main conclusions. First, Islam and its institutional forms do impact ethical decision-making in the day-to-day practice of biomedical research in countries with a Muslim population and/or in the research careers of Muslim researchers. Secondly, it shows that there are many distinctive mechanisms, such as the involvement of Islamic scholars, the process of ijtihad (independent reasoning) and the production of *fatawah* (legal edicts), by which Islam identifies and develops ethical views about biomedical matters. Thirdly, HIV/AIDS poses major challenges to the world of Islam as it does the rest of world. The epidemic raises issues that touch on cultural sensitivities that are important to Islamic societies, and this study has shown that no simple or single response was observed to the ethical issues arising from HIV/AIDS. Fourthly, researchers face practical challenges when deliberating women's autonomy in contexts where Islam is appropriated within "male dominated" contexts. The role and status of women is disputed in such contexts, with views ranging from women needing their husbands' permission to leave the home to men and women having equal freedoms. Fifth and finally, this study describes and analyses how the personal faith of researchers and their deep commitment to Islamic ethics and law influences their understanding of their legal and moral accountability and ethico-legal decision-making. It shows that researchers adopt multiple roles and are required to balance numerous value systems and priorities.

They face moral anxiety and frustration when these different moral sources are in conflict. Overall, this study indicates that, in the countries studied, Islam does influence biomedical research ethics, and that this can be appreciated through the growing reference to Islam and its scriptural sources in biomedical research ethics literature, research ethics guidelines and the role of Islam in the day-to-day practice of biomedical researchers in the case study sites, which has been captured in the empirical study.

Chapter 8 – This chapter outlines in detail the rationale and method for the empirical study as well as study limitations. It presents how study sites were chosen, data collection instruments were designed, and data was collected and analysed. The chapter also presents the various advantages and disadvantages of the methods considered to enable the reader to understand why the chosen method was employed.

Bibliography

Adamson, P. (2015). *Philosophy in the Islamic world: A very short introduction.* Oxford: Oxford University Press.

Alahmad, G., Al-Jumah, M. & Dierickx, K. (2012). Review of national research ethics regulations and guidelines in middle eastern Arab countries. *BMC Medical Ethics,* 13(1). doi:10.1186/1472-6939-13-34.

Al-Bar, M. A. & Chamsi-Pasha, H. (2015). *Contemporary bioethics: Islamic perspective.* New York: Springer.

Annas, G. J. & Grodin, M. A. (2008). The Nuremberg Code. In E. J. Emanuel, C. C. Grady, R. A. Crouch, R. K. Lie & F. G. Miller (Eds.). *The Oxford textbook of clinical research ethics.* (pp. 136–140). New York: Oxford University Press.

Bagheri, A. (2014). Priority setting in Islamic bioethics: Top 10 bioethical challenges in Islamic countries. *Asian Bioethics Review,* 6(4), 391–401. doi:10.1353/asb.2014.0031.

Berlinguer, G. (2004). Bioethics, health, and inequality. *The Lancet,* 364(9439), 1086–1091. doi:10.1016/s0140-6736(04)17066-9.

Bhutta, Z. A. (2002). Ethics in international health research: A perspective from the developing world. *Bulletin of the World Health Organization,* 80(2), 114–120.

Blum, L. A. (1994). *Moral perception and particularity.* Cambridge: Cambridge University Press.

Bracanovic, T. (2010). Respect for cultural diversity in bioethics: Empirical, conceptual and normative constraints. *Medicine, Health Care and Philosophy,* 14(3), 229–236. doi:10.1007/s11019-010-9299-3.

Brockopp, J. E. & Eich, T. (2008). *Muslim medical ethics: From theory to practice.* Columbia, SC: University of South Carolina Press.

Caballero, B. (2002). Ethical issues for collaborative research in developing countries. *The American Journal of Clinical Nutrition,* 76(4), 717–720.

Chattopadhyay, S. & De Vries, R. (2012). Respect for cultural diversity in bioethics is an ethical imperative. *Medicine, Health Care and Philosophy,* 16(4), 639–645. doi:10.1007/s11019-012-9433-5.

Clausen, C. (1996). Welcome to post-culturalism. *The American Scholar,* 65(3), 379–388.

Curran, W. J. (1973). The Tuskegee syphilis study. *New England Journal of Medicine,* 289 (14), 730–731. doi:10.1056/nejm197310042891406.

Dancy, J. (2004). *Ethics without principles*. Oxford: Oxford University Press on Demand.

Dawson, C. (2013). *Religion and culture*. Washington, DC: CUA Press.

Dunn, M., Sheehan, M., Hope, T. & Parker, M. (2012). Toward methodological innovation in empirical ethics research. *Cambridge Quarterly of Healthcare Ethics*, 21(04), 466–480.

Durante, C. (2008). Bioethics in a pluralistic society: Bioethical methodology in lieu of moral diversity. *Medicine, Health Care and Philosophy*, 12(1), 35–47. doi:10.1007/s11019-008-9148-9.

El Fadl, K. A. (2014). *Speaking in God's name: Islamic law, authority and women*. Oxford: Oneworld Publications.

Emanuel, E. J., Wendler, D. & Grady, C. (2000). What makes clinical research ethical? *JAMA*, 283(20), 2701–2711.

Emanuel, E. J., Wendler, D., Killen, J. & Grady, C. (2004). What makes clinical research in developing countries ethical?: The benchmarks of ethical research. *The Journal of Infectious Diseases*, 189(5), 930–937. doi:10.1086/381709.

Fakhry, M. (1991). *Ethical theories in Islam* (8). Leiden, The Netherlands: Brill.

Fakhry, M. (2009). *Islamic philosophy: A beginner's guide*. London: Oneworld Publications.

Freedman, B. (1987). Scientific value and validity as ethical requirements for research: A proposed explication. *IRB: Ethics and Human Research*, 9(6), 7–10. doi:10.2307/3563623.

Frieden, T. R. & Collins, F. S. (2010). Intentional infection of vulnerable populations in 1946–1948. *JAMA*, 304(18), 2063–2064. doi:10.1001/jama.2010.1554.

Garrafa, V., Solbakk, J. H., Vidal, S. & Lorenzo, C. (2010). Between the needy and the greedy: The quest for a just and fair ethics of clinical research. *Journal of Medical Ethics*, 36(8), 500–504. doi:10.1136/jme.2009.032656.

Garrard, E. & Wilkinson, S. (2005). Mind the gap: The use of empirical evidence in bioethics. In M. Häyry, T. Takala & P. Herissone-Kelly (Eds.). *Bioethics and social reality* (pp. 77–92). Amsterdam, The Netherlands: Rodopi.

Gatrad, A. R. & Sheikh, A. (2001). Medical ethics and Islam: Principles and practice. *Archives of Disease in Childhood*, 84(1), 72–75.

Ghaly, M. (2013a). Collective religio-scientific discussions on Islam and HIV/AIDS: I. Biomedical scientists. *Zygon®*, 48(3), 671–708.

Global Forum for Health Research (2004). *The 10/90 report on health research, 2003–2004*. Switzerland: Global Forum for Health Research.

Hallaq, W. B. (2009). *Shari'a: Theory, practice, transformations*. Cambridge: Cambridge University Press.

Hodgson, M. G. S. (1977a). *The venture of Islam: Conscience and history in a world Civilization. Volume 1: The classical age of Islam*. Chicago, IL: University of Chicago Press.

Ibn Majah. Book 31, Hadith 3436. *Sunan Ibn Majah*. http://sunnah.com/ibnmajah/31 (Last accessed 23 August 2016).

IJsselmuiden, C. B., Kass, N. E., Sewankambo, K. N. & Lavery, J. V. (2010). Evolving values in ethics and global health research. *Global Public Health*, 5(2), 154–163. doi:10.1080/17441690903436599.

Ilkilic, I. (2002). Bioethical conflicts between Muslim patients and German physicians and the principles of biomedical ethics. *Med. & L.*, 21(2), 243–256.

Inhorn, M. C. (2008). Conclusion. In J. E. Brockopp & T. Eich (Eds.). *Muslim medical ethics: From theory to practice* (pp. 252–256). Columbia, SC: University of South Carolina Press.

Inhorn, M. C. (2012). *Local babies, global science: Gender, religion and in vitro fertilization in Egypt*. New York: Routledge.

Inhorn, M. C. & Serour, G. I. (2011). Islam, medicine, and Arab-Muslim refugee health in America after 9/11. *The Lancet*, 378(9794), 935–943. doi:10.1016/s0140-6736(11) 61041-6.

Ives, J. & Dunn, M. (2010). Who's arguing?: A call for reflexivity in bioethics. *Bioethics*, 24 (5), 256–265.

Ives, J., Dunn, M. & Cribb, A. (Eds.). (2016). *Empirical bioethics: Theoretical and practical perspectives* (Vol. 37). Cambridge: Cambridge University Press.

Jonsen, A. R. (1998). *The birth of bioethics*. Oxford: Oxford University Press.

Kazim, F. (2007). Critical analysis of the Pakistan Medical Dental Council code and bioethical issues. Master's Thesis in Applied Ethics. Linköpings universitet, Sweden. Centre for Applied Ethics. Presented June 2007. http://www.diva-portal.org/smash/get/diva 2:23919/FULLTEXT01.pdf (Last accessed 29 April 2016).

Kon, A. A. (2009). The role of empirical research in bioethics. *The American Journal of Bioethics*, 9(6–7), 59–65. doi:10.1080/15265160902874320.

Kyriakides-Yeldham, A. (2005). Islamic medical ethics and the straight path of God. *Islam and Christian–Muslim Relations*, 16(3), 213–225.

Leget, C., Borry, P. & De Vries, R. (2009). "Nobody Tosses a Dwarf!": The relation between the empirical and the normative reexamined. *Bioethics*, 23(4), 226–235.

Lin, V. (1997). Resource review. Investing in health research and development: Report of the ad hoc committee on health research relating to future intervention options. World Health Organization, Geneva, 1996. *Health Promotion International*, 12(4), 331–332. doi:10.1093/heapro/12.4.331.

Lings, M. (2012). *Muhammad: His life based on the earliest sources*. Cambridge: Islamic Texts Society.

Lurie, P. & Wolfe, S. M. (1997). Unethical trials of interventions to reduce perinatal transmission of the human immunodeficiency virus in developing countries. *New England Journal of Medicine*, 337(12), 853–856. doi:10.1056/nejm199709183371212.

Macklin, R. (1999). *Against relativism: Cultural diversity and the search for ethical universals in medicine*. New York: Oxford University Press.

Mālik, A. Book 47, no. 47.1.8. *Al-Muwatta of Imam Malik ibn Anas: The first formulation of Islamic law*. http://ahadith.co.uk/chapter.php?cid=97 (Last accessed 23 August 2016).

Nuffield Council on Bioethics. (2002). *The ethics of research related to healthcare in developing countries*. London: Nuffield Council on Bioethics.

Padela, A. I. (2013a). Islamic bioethics: Between sacred law, lived experiences, and state authority. *Theoretical Medicine and Bioethics*, 34(2), 65–80. doi:10.1007/s11017-013-9249-1.

Padela, A. I. & Punekar, I. R. A. (2009). Emergency medical practice: Advancing cultural competence and reducing health care disparities. *Academic Emergency Medicine*, 16(1), 69–75. doi:10.1111/j.1553-2712.2008.00305.x.

Parker, M. (2012). *Ethical problems and genetics practice*. Cambridge: Cambridge University Press.

Plato (1914). *Plato: Euthyphro, Apology, Crito, Phaedo, Phaedrus* (H. N. Fowler, Trans.). Cambridge, MA: The Loeb Classical Library. Harvard University Press.

Ramadan, T. (2009). *Radical reform: Islamic ethics and liberation*. New York: Oxford University Press.

Raysuni, A. (2005). *Imam al-Shatibi's theory of the higher objectives and intents of Islamic law*. London: International Institute of Islamic Thought.

Ryan, M. A. (2004). Beyond a Western bioethics? *Theological Studies*, 65(1), 158–177. doi:10.1177/004056390406500105.

Sachedina, A. (2009). *Islamic biomedical ethics: Principles and application*. New York: Oxford University Press.

Sachedina, A. & Ainuddin, N. (2004). *Islamic biomedical ethics: Issues and resources*. Islamabad: COMSTECH.

Sartell, E. & Padela, A. I. (2015). Adab and its significance for an Islamic medical ethics. *Journal of Medical Ethics*, 41(9), 756–761. doi:10.1136/medethics-2014-102276.

Shabana, A. (2013). Religious and cultural legitimacy of bioethics: Lessons from Islamic bioethics. *Medicine, Health Care and Philosophy*, 16(4), 671–677. doi:10.1007/s11019-013-9472-6.

Siddiqui, A. (1997). Ethics in Islam: Key concepts and contemporary challenges. *Journal of Moral Education*, 26(4), 423–431. doi:10.1080/0305724970260403.

Silverman, H. (Ed.). (2017). *Research ethics in the Arab region*. Cham, Switzerland: Springer International Publishing.

Singer, P. (Ed.). (1994). *Ethics*. Oxford: Oxford University Press.

Sleem, H., El-Kamary, S. S. & Silverman, H. J. (2010). Identifying structures, processes, resources and needs of research ethics committees in Egypt. *BMC Medical Ethics*, 11 (12). doi:10.1186/1472-6939-11-12.

Suleman, M. (2016). Contributions and ambiguities in Islamic research ethics and research conducted in Muslim contexts: I – A thematic review of the literature. *Journal of Health and Culture* 1(1): 46–57.

Syed, I. B. (1981). Islamic medicine: 1000 years ahead of its times. *Journal of the Islamic Medical Association of North America*, 13(1). doi:10.5915/13-1-11925.

ten Have, H. (2013). Global bioethics: Transnational experiences and Islamic bioethics. *Zygon®*, 48(3), 600–617.

ten Have, H. & Gordijn, B. (2010). Travelling bioethics. *Medicine, Health Care and Philosophy*, 14(1), 1–3. doi:10.1007/s11019-010-9300-1.

Tremayne, S. (2009). Law, ethics and donor technologies in Shia Iran. In D. Birenbaum-Carmeli & M. C. Inhorn (Eds.). *Assisting reproduction, testing genes: Global encounters with the new Biotechnologies* (pp. 144–163). Oxford: Berghahn Books.

Weindling, P. (2008). The Nazi medical experiments. In E. J. Emanuel (Ed.). *The Oxford textbook of clinical research ethics* (pp. 18–30). Oxford: Oxford University Press.

Widdershoven, G., Hope, T. & McMillan, J. (Eds.). (2008). *Empirical ethics in psychiatry*. Oxford: Oxford University Press.

Winter, T. (Ed.). (2008). *The Cambridge companion to classical Islamic theology* (3rd ed.). Cambridge: Cambridge University Press.

Winter, T. J. & Williams, J. A. (2003). *Understanding Islam and the Muslims: Expanded to include the Muslim family and Islam and world peace*. Louisville, KY: Fons Vitae of Kentucky.

Yusuf, A. (2014). Ethical issues in research ethics governance and their application to the Malaysian context. DPhil thesis. University of Oxford.

Zahedi, F., Emami Razavi, S. H. & Larijani, B. (2009). A two-decade review of medical ethics in Iran. *Iranian J Publ Health*, 38(Suppl 1), 40–46.

2 Guideline review

Why is a guideline search and review necessary?

Research and writings on ethical issues arising from human subject research, within the Islamic tradition, dates back to the medieval period. For example, *Ibn Sina* articulated the need for research on humans when he wrote that "the experimentation must be done with [the] human body, for testing a drug on a lion or a horse might not prove anything about its effect on man" (Sachedina, 2009, p. 197). However, a systematic establishment of ethical guidelines and committees to oversee research practices in Muslim countries is a recent phenomenon. This is partly due to the recent rise in biomedical research within Muslim countries (Alahmad et al., 2012), the need to comply with contemporary international ethical standards and also recognition from organisations such as IOMS of the need to establish an "Islamic viewpoint" on the ethics of clinical research (Fadel, 2010). The latter involved a meeting of biomedical experts and Muslim scholars in Kuwait in 2006, which resulted in a publication providing an Islamic perspective on international ethical principles and guidelines (Fadel, 2010).

Although studies have been conducted to assess the ethical protocols within Arab countries (Alahmad et al., 2012; Silverman 2017) no work has been done to comprehensively review ethical guidelines throughout the Muslim world, nor has an analysis been made of these guidelines to assess how they incorporate Islamic values, if at all. This chapter is a review of the clinical research documents submitted within the OIC (Organisation of Islamic Cooperation), which has been taken to represent the "Muslim world". Malaysia helped establish the OIC in 1969. It is comprised of 57 countries and has headquarters in Jeddah, Saudi Arabia. The organisation was formed to promote cooperation between countries with an Islamic identity. It identifies its mandate as: "the collective voice of the Muslim world and ensuring to safeguard and protect the interests of the Muslim world in the spirit of promoting international peace and harmony among various people of the world".[1] The organisation's mandate has been extended to embrace cooperation in the matter of health also.[2] This chapter will focus on reviewing the

---

1 Organisation of Islamic Cooperation. http://www.oic-oci.org/oicv3/page/?p_id=52&p_ref=26&lan=en (Last accessed 4 January 2014).
2 Organisation of Islamic Cooperation. http://www.oic-oci.org (Last accessed 4 January 2014).

extent to which ethical protections are offered, in the guidelines found, and establishing the role, if any, that the Islamic tradition, through the normative texts and associated scholarship, plays within the national/regional/international discourses on research ethics, in informing ethical decision-making.

Methods of guideline search and review

Data collection

A range of data collection methods were employed, including direct access to governmental agency websites, ministries of health, food and drug administrations (FDAs), medical councils, research centres and national committees of bioethics in the 57 OIC countries. It also included examination of the Office for Human Research Protections (OHRP) database,[3] emailing ministries of health for guidelines, consulting an existing paper that reviewed 13 Arab states (Alahmad et al., 2012), as well as a Google search for each of the 57 OIC countries.

My study selection included all national and/or institutional codes or guidelines, sourced by contacting the ministries of health via email or consulting available online resources that addressed research ethics either exclusively or partially. The guideline search strategy is displayed in Table 2.1.

The data collated from the searches was initially stored and analysed using Excel. The following headings were used for the initial storing and charting of data/links:[4]

- Is country listed on OHRP?
- Are the OHRP guidelines accessible?
- Are there guidelines through the MoH?
- Or other government sources?
- Guideline link
- Do the guidelines deal with clinical research?
- Do the guidelines contain reference to Islam and/or Muslims?
- If yes, then to what extent?
- Other
- Local/other contact (email address/telephone)

Method of reviewing the guidelines and ethical protections stated in the research ethics documents for 17 OIC countries

After reviewing 57 countries, 24 documents were found from 18 countries. These documents were studied considering the ethical principles stated in the

---

3 Office for Human Research Protections (OHRP). (2014). http://www.hhs.gov/ohrp/ (Last accessed 1 December 2014).
4 Personal email addresses were included in the table, however, without individual permissions being issued, they have not been reproduced here.

Table 2.1 Guideline search strategy

Data source	Search method	Results	Date of search	Additional notes
Google search	Free text search: "Research ethics guidelines Islam Muslim"	1,580,000	20/3/2014	Search did not yield any specific guidelines. However, the following references were found: 1. WHO (2005). This was produced in conjunction with IOMS – there were no specific reference to "research" or "research ethics" other than to the work IOMS has done to produce guidelines on an Islamic perspective on research ethics. 2. Alahmad et al. (2012) reference also found – may be a useful source of guidelines
Search for IOMS guideline				
Google search	Free text search: "IOMS research ethics"	4,313	20/3/2014	Not able to locate the IOMS guideline through this search
Google search	Free text search: "IOMS Islamic perspective research ethics"	67,340	20/3/2014	Not able to locate the IOMS guideline through this search
IOMS website	Direct browsing of website to find guideline	1	20/3/2014	Islamic Organization of Medical Sciences (2014). Text found different to that referenced in Fadel (2010)
Google Search	Free text	1	20/3/2014	Link found via Georgetown University to a PDF version of the IOMS guideline CIOMS (2002). The PDF is legible, however, again the text is different to that referenced in Fadel (2010)

Email to IOMS email	Email sent re: version of IOMS guidelines and whether I could be sent a copy of the different versions	20/3/2014	No reply
Email sent to IOMS member	Meeting with IOMS member in Jordan November 2014.	1	26/1/2015	I mentioned to her my DPhil project and the difficulty in obtaining a hard copy of the IOMS guidelines. She took my postal address and agreed to post me a copy. The hard copy of the guidelines was received 26 January 2015. This version confirmed the text found in Fadel (2010).

Search for guidelines from Alahmad et al. (2012)

Alahmad et al. (2012)	List of references from the paper	10	20/3/2014	These are all complete and accessible online from the paper.

Search from OHRP database

http://www.hhs.gov/ohrp/	List of guidelines from the OHRP corresponding with OIC countries	11	21/3/2014	The OHRP database listed the following: 22 OIC countries 11 accessible guidelines

Search for guidelines from governmental agency websites

Google search of OIC countries -Medical councils -FDAs -MoH - Research centres - National committees of bioethics	Direct browsing of websites			See Table 2.2

(Continued)

Table 2.1 (Cont.)

Data source	Search method	Results	Date of search	Additional notes
Search for guidelines via emailing				
Email sent to ministries with addresses listed online or found on published reports/documents				See table below
Other searches				
Search for Grey literature using "Open Grey" http://www.opengrey.eu	Free text search for "research ethics guidelines" "ethics guidelines"	0 15 – no results applicable to this study	22/3/2014	No results found No results related to the OIC countries – ethical guidelines found from the UK RCP (http://www.opengrey.eu/item/display/10068/424632) and the Paediatric Association (http://www.opengrey.eu/item/display/10068/441133)

Declaration of Helsinki, the Council for International Organizations of Medical Sciences (CIOMS) (2002) guidelines and the International Conference of Harmonization – Guidelines for Good Clinical Practice (ICH-GCP). The rationale for this was in keeping with the work of Alahmad et al. (2012), who explain:

> Owing to their wide acceptance around the world, we selected the Declaration of Helsinki and the ICH-GCP for comparison. We selected the CIOMS guidelines for the same reason, but also because they were crafted specifically with the aim of applying the Declaration of Helsinki to developing countries in a way that reflects the conditions and needs of biomedical research in those countries, and due to the implications for the multinational or transnational research in which they may be partners. A list of 19 ethical protections taken from these international documents was used in our comparison.
>
> (p. 2)

I have used the same list of 19 ethical protections to critically review the 24 documents and to assess what protections they offer in order to compare them with the international guidelines.

All relevant documents in English, or the available translations of documents in Arabic or French, were included in the study.

Analysing the role of Islam within research guidelines

Within the review of the 24 documents, references to Islam and Islamic sources (the normative texts, scholarship and the subsequent interpretation and derived sciences) and Muslim religio-cultural influences were searched for and analysed to ascertain whether these were used as a reference within the content of the guidelines and, if so, to what extent. The mention of a particular theme was recorded. However, the frequency of occurrence was not recorded. For example, the use of *Quranic* references and mention of *Hadith* or issues around female consent may have been mentioned multiple times in one guideline, however, these were noted as a simple tick in Table 2.4. A more detailed description of how the themes are mentioned in the guidelines is discussed below.

Findings of guideline search and review

Twenty-one countries were found to have ethics laws and/or guidelines that mention research. Three countries, Morocco, Algeria and the Kyrgyz Republic, were excluded, as the documents found were not available in English. Attempts were made to contact guideline authors and publishing organisations in order to request English translations. However, no reply was received. Without officially approved translations, these documents were not included. English translations of documents that were used from other countries had official approval from issuing organisations, such as the ministries of health, research ethics committees, etc. In order to ensure that the documents included within this analysis were in keeping with nationally approved translation and publication practices, guidelines that did not meet these criteria were excluded. It was also not feasible to wait for official translations to be published given the time constraints of the research period. Reviewing the 18 remaining countries yielded 24 documents, and these were analysed. Table 2.2 lists the guidelines that were found. Those highlighted in grey were not available in English, and those italicised (e.g., some of the guidelines listed for Indonesia) were not found.

Tables 2.3a–2.3c display the 24 documents against the 19 ethical protections from the international documents mentioned above. Of the 18 countries reviewed, different levels and kinds of research ethics laws and guidelines were found. There were three overall levels: (1) there is detailed mention of ethical protections within research, (2) there is a nominal mention and (3) there are no guidelines yet established. The majority of the documents that were assessed refer to one or more international guidelines on bioethics. Of the guidelines reviewed, the ethics code of Qatar had the highest number of protections at 17, and Indonesia had the least with two. The elements most commonly cited include informed consent and the need for ethics committee review. The elements least cited include research with limited resources and the obligation to provide healthcare.

Tables 2.3a–2.3c also highlight the areas where differences were noted with Alhamad et al.'s (2012) analysis. Review of the Kuwait guideline revealed that there is mention of confidentiality on page five.[5] When reviewing the Lebanon guideline, consent by parents or a legal representative is stated as necessary for minors and those incapacitated.[6] The review of the Qatar guideline, revealed that there was neither mention of research with limited resources nor obligation to provide healthcare.[7] The Saudi Arabian guideline "The Law of ethics of research on living creatures" does mention the need to inform research participants of the risks and potential outcomes of the trial.[8] The Saudi Arabia guideline "Ethics of the medical profession" mentions of the objectives of research, including the "enriching" of medical knowledge.[9] In the UAE guideline,

---

5   Kuwait Institute of Medical Specialities (KIMS). (2009). Ethical guidelines for biomedical research. http://www.kims.org.kw/Ethical%202.doc (Last accessed June 2014).

6   Code of medical ethics: Free translation from Arabic. Law no. 240 dated October 22, 2012, amending law no. 288 of February 22, 1994. (2012). http://www.aub.edu.lb/fm/shbpp/ethics/public/Documents/New-Code-of-Medical-Ethics-text-ENGLISH.pdf (Last accessed June 2014).

7   Qatar Supreme Council of Health. (2009). Guidelines, regulations and policies for research involving human subjects. http://qatar-weill.cornell.edu/research/pdf/Ministry%20Guidelines.doc (Last accessed June 2014).

8   Law of ethics of research on living creatures. Issued under Royal decree no. M/59 dated 14.9.1431 AH, Ministerial resolution no. 321 dated 13.9.1431 AH and Circular of the Minister of Justice no. 13/T/4202 dated 3.4.1432 AH. (2014). http://old.sfda.gov.sa/NR/rdonlyres/D6892236-AF58-41B2-9AC4-DE0E3BF53380/0/ClinicalTrialsRequirmentsGuidelines_12.pdf (Last accessed June 2014).

9   Saudi Council for Health Specialists. (2014). Ethics of the medical profession. http://dent.ksu.edu.sa/sites/default/files/rr/35.pdf (Last accessed June 2014).

Table 2.2 Research ethics guidelines found in 21 OIC countries – Guidelines for 18 countries available in English

Country	Entity	Year	Guideline	Guideline description	Guideline link (last accessed June 2014)
People's Demo-cratic Republic of Algeria	*Needs translating – currently available in French*				http://www.news.clinpower.com/wp-content/uploads/2011/02/ALger-ianLawOnClinicalTrials.pdf
Kingdom of Bahrain	Ministry of Health	2009	Ethical guidelines for health research (within the document titled "Health research structure & processes")	One A4 side	http://www.moh.gov.bh/PDF/Health%20Research%20Structure%20and%20Proce-dures%20%20DRAFT.pdf
Bangladesh	Medical Research Council	2013	National research ethics guideline	89 pages	PDF received from info@bmrcbd.org
Brunei Darussalam					Email received that committee adopts WHO guidelines
Arab Republic of Egypt	Ministry of Health and Population	2003	Professional ethics regulations no. 238 – Specific section titled "Conducting medical research & experiments on human beings"	2.5 A4 sides	http://www.cms.org.eg/user-files/file/kanon/leha_eng.doc; http://ec.europa.eu/bepa/eur-opean-group-ethics/docs/ibd/lamis_ragab_(egypt).ppt

(Continued)

Table 2.2 (Cont.)

Country	Entity	Year	Guideline	Guideline description	Guideline link (last accessed June 2014)
Indonesia	Ministry of Health	1992; 2002; 2004; 2009; *Those italicised were not found*	Indonesian health act no. 23/1992 section on health research, article 69; *Regulation no. 1333/2002 agreement on human research, No.1334/2002, regarding national ethics committee on health research; National ethics guidelines on health research ministerial decree no. 657/Menkes/PER/8/2009 Regarding guideline sending the specimen for health's R & D*		Email received that committee use the Nuremberg Code, the Declaration of Helsinki, the CIOMS International Guidelines for Biomedical Research Involving Human Subjects, and the Belmont Report as their main international references
Islamic Republic of Iran	Iran's Ministry of Health and Medical Education	1999–2000	Protection code of human subject in medical research	26 codes; 1.5 A4 sides	http://emrc.tums.ac.ir/upfiles/91710105.pdf

Country	Authority	Year	Document	Details	URL
Hashemite Kingdom of Jordan	Prime Minister's Council	2001	Law of clinical studies: Provisional law no. 97 for 2001	17 Articles; 8 A4 sides	http://www.jfda.jo/Download/Laws/32_139.doc; http://www.jfda.jo/Download/Laws/33_131.doc
Kyrgyz Republic	*Needs translating – currently available in Kyrgyz*		Health protection act; Law on drugs; Rules on clinical testing of medical products		
State of Kuwait	Kuwait Institute of Medical Specialisation (KIMS) of the Ministry of Health	2009	Ethical guidelines for biomedical research	18 A4 sides; Draft consent form; Information for participants; Evaluation form	http://www.kims.org.kw/Ethical%202.doc
Republic of Lebanon	Parliamentary Council of Lebanon	1994; amendments 2012;	Law of medical ethics no. 288	Section on "Human experiments, transplants, artificial insemination and abortion" –Human experimentation covered by article 30 – one A4 side	http://www.aub.edu.lb/fm/shbpp/ethics/public/Documents/New-Code-of-Medical-Ethics-text-ENGLISH.pdf; http://f-mri.org/upload/2011–2012/Lebanese_MOH_Directive_for_clinical_trials__Jan_2012__guidelines.pdf
Kingdom of Morocco	*Needs translating – currently available in French*				http://pharmacies.ma/pharmacie/imprimer.php?module=textes_de_loi&name=dahir_centres_hospitaliers

(*Continued*)

Table 2.2 (Cont.)

Country	Entity	Year	Guideline	Guideline description	Guideline link (last accessed June 2014)
Malaysia	National Committee for Clinical Research; Malaysian Medical Council	2011; 2006	Malaysian guide for good clinical practice; Clinical trials and biomedical research	94 pages; 32 pages	http://www.nccr.gov.my/view_file.cfm?fileid=3; http://mmc.gov.my/v1/docs/Clinical%20Trials%20%20&%20Biomedical%20Research.pdf
Federal Republic of Nigeria	Federal Ministry of Health	2007	National code of health research ethics	56 pages	http://nhrec.net/nhrec/download-nchre
Sultanate of Oman	Research and Ethical Review and Approve Committee	No date	Guidelines for research proposal to be submitted for review, approval and registration	10 A4 sides	http://www.moh.gov.om/en/rec/Guideline_for_research_proposal.pdf
Islamic Republic of Pakistan	The Pakistan Medical and Dental Council; National Bioethics Committee Pakistan	2001	Code of ethics for medical and dental practitioners; Ethical research committee guidelines	20 pages; 5 pages	http://www.pmdc.org.pk/Ethics/tabid/101/Default.aspx#1; http://www.pmrc.org.pk/erc_guidelines.htm
State of Qatar	Qatar Supreme Council of Health	2009	Guidelines, regulations and policies for research involving human subjects;	24 pages	http://qatar-weill.cornell.edu/research/pdf/Ministry%20Guidelines.doc

| Kingdom of Saudi Arabia | Saudi Food and Drug Authority; Royal Decree – circular of ministry of justice; Saudi Council for Health Specialties; National committee of bioethics | 2008; 2009; 1997; 2010 | Clinical trials requirement guidelines; The law of ethics of research on living creatures; Ethics of the medical profession; Implementing regulations of the law of ethics on research on living creatures | 65 pages; 8 pages; 32 pages; 109 pages | http://old.sfda.gov.sa/NR/rdonlyres/E3752369-0065-49A0-AACA-08DACBF16262/0/التجاربالاكلينيكية |
| Republic of The Sudan | National Ministry of Health | 2008 | National guidelines for ethical conduct of research involving human subjects | 80 pages | أخلاقياتالتجاربعلى.pdf; http://old.sfda.gov.sa/NR/rdonlyres/D689 2236-AF58-41B2-9AC4-DE0E3BF53380/0/ClinicalTrialsRequirmentsGuidelines_12.pdf; http://dent.ksu.edu.sa/sites/default/files/rr/35.pdf; http://adl.moj.gov.sa/ENG/attach/228.pdf; http://www.kacst.edu.sa/ar/depts/bioethics/Documents/The%20final%20draft%20of%20the%20translation%20Law%20and%20Regulations2.pdf https://www.healthresearchweb.org/files/Final%20national%20ethical%20guidelines-last%20draft.pdf |

(*Continued*)

Table 2.2 (Cont.)

Country	Entity	Year	Guideline	Guideline description	Guideline link (last accessed June 2014)
Republic of Turkey	Ministry of Health	2011	Regulation on clinical trials	20 pages online	http://www.iegm.gov.tr/Default.aspx?sayfa=regulations&lang=en&tthelawtype=148&tthelawId=398
State of The United Arab Emirates	Ministry of Health	2006	Guidance for conducting clinical trials based on drugs/medicinal products and good clinical practice		http://www.cpd-pharma.ae/index.php?option=com_phocadownload&view=category&download=16:h-uac-gcp-guide-2006-english&id=1:pdf-files&Itemid=63
Republic of Uganda	Ministry of Health; National Drug Authority; Uganda National Council for Science and Technology	2008; 2007	National Drug Authority guidelines for the conduct of clinical trials; National guidelines for research involving humans as research participants	22 pages; 50 pages	http://apps.who.int/medicinedocs/documents/s19724en/s19724en.pdf; http://www.unist.go.ug/dmdocuments/Guideline,%20Human%20Subjects%20Guidelines%20Marc.pdf

information to be included during the consent process is listed, and the review of external sponsors is detailed.[10]

Mention of Islam as a reference in the research ethics documents for 19 OIC countries

Of the 18 countries that do have guidelines, ten of the 24 guidelines mention Islam, Islamic sources or the Muslim religio-cultural context. These ten guidelines are from eight countries. Tables 2.3a–2.3c summarize the country guidelines that contain such details and list the themes within which Islam, its sources and the Muslim religio-cultural influence appear within the guidelines. Those highlighted in grey have no mention of Islam.

Discussion

The review in this chapter has involved an analysis of the current research protocols, guidelines and laws submitted within the OIC to primarily assess the underlying normative principles that govern and inform local ethical decision-making and to compare these with global ethical principles. Although studies have been conducted to assess the ethical protocols within a few Arab countries (Alahmad et al., 2012; Silverman, 2017), no work has been done to comprehensively review ethical guidelines throughout the OIC, nor has an analysis been made of these guidelines to assess how they incorporate Islamic values, if at all.

Wide variation in presence of guidelines or laws and levels of protections

Despite global efforts to raise awareness of ethical challenges encountered within research and methods to counter these, the majority of the countries within the OIC are yet to establish guidelines, protocols or laws relating to human subject research. The review shows that of the 21 countries that do have guidelines, many are within the wealthy Gulf States. Alahmad et al., (2012) have noted that this may be because of greater investments being made by the Gulf Cooperation Council (GCC) countries into healthcare and research. In addition to the GCC states investing in the establishment of their own research institutes and funding local research, resource-poor countries like Sudan and Uganda have also established guidelines. The latter may have done so as they are common sites for international research, and local ethical guidelines and research ethics committees are considered a necessity by many international funders and research institutions.

---

10 UAE Ministry of Health. (2006). Guidance for conducting clinical trials based on drugs/medicinal products and good clinical practice. http://www.cpdpharma.ae/index.php?option=com_phocadownload&view=category&download=16:huae-gcp-guide-2006-english&id=1:pdf-files&Itemid=63 (Last accessed June 2014).

Table 2.3a Ethical protections stated in 24 documents of 18 OIC Countries

19 Protections	Frequency of Protections	Kingdom of Bahrain — Ethical guidelines for health research	Bangladesh — National research ethics guideline	Arab Republic of Egypt — Professional ethics regulations	Indonesia — Health Act no. 23/1992 section on health research, Article 69	Islamic Republic of Iran — Protection code of the human subject in research	Jordan — Law of clinical studies	Kuwait — Ethical guidelines for biomedical research	Lebanon — Law of medical ethics
Informed consent	23	✓	✓	✓	✗	✓	✓	✓	✓
E. C.	22	✓	✓	✓	✗	✓	✓	✓	✓
Scientific validity	19	✓	✓	✓	✓	✗	✓	✓	✗
Confidentiality	20	✓	✓	✓	✗	✓	✗	✓	✗
Benefits and risks of participation	20	✓	✓	✓	✓	✓	✗	✓	✗
Limitations of risk of research on incapables	11	✗	✗	✓	✗	✓	✗	✗	✗
Inducement to participate	14	✗	✓	✗	✗	✓	✗	✓	✗
Consent of incapables	15	✗	✓	✓	✗	✓	✗	✗	✓
Research involving children	16	✗	✓	✓	✗	✓	✗	✗	✓

Ethical review of externally sponsored research	9	✓	✓	✗	✗	✗	✗	✗
Information in the I.C.	11	✗	✓	✗	✗	✗	✓	✗
Who is responsible for collecting the I.C.	8	✗	✗	✗	✗	✓	✓	✗
Research with limited resources	1	✗	✗	✗	✗	✗	✗	✗
Research involving vulnerable persons	13	✗	✓	✓	✓	✓	✗	✗
Compensation	12	✗	✓	✗	✗	✗	✗	✗
Strengthening ethical and scientific capacity	9	✗	✓	✗	✗	✗	✗	✗
Obligation to provide healthcare	5	✗	✓	✗	✗	✗	✗	✗
Women as research subjects	7	✗	✓	✗	✗	✗	✗	✗

(Continued)

Table 2.3a (Cont.)

19 Protections	Frequency of Protections	Kingdom of Bahrain	Bangladesh	Arab Republic of Egypt	Indonesia	Islamic Republic of Iran	Jordan	Kuwait	Lebanon
		Ethical guidelines for health research	National research ethics guideline	Professional ethics regulations	Health Act no. 23/1992 section on health research, Article 69	Protection code of the human subject in research	Law of clinical studies	Ethical guidelines for biomedical research	Law of medical ethics
Equitable distribution of burdens and benefits	6	x	✓	x	x	x	x	x	x
Total number of protections		8	16	9	2	10	3	8	4

Key: ✓ = Protection present
x = Protection absent

Different result to Alahmad et al. (2012)

Abbreviations:
I.C. = Informed consent
E.C. = Ethics committee

Table 2.3b Ethical protections stated in 24 documents of 18 OIC Countries

19 Protections	Frequency of Protections	Malaysia — Malaysian guideline for good clinical practice	Malaysia — Guideline of the MMC – clinical trials and bio-medical research	Nigeria — National code of health research ethics	Oman — Guidelines for research proposal to be submitted for review	Pakistan — Code of ethics for medical and dental practitioners	Pakistan — Ethical research committee guidelines	Qatar — Guidelines, regulations and policies for research involving human subjects
Informed consent	23	✓	✓	✓	✓	✓	✓	✓
E. C.	22	✓	✓	✓	x	✓	✓	✓
Scientific validity	19	✓	✓	✓	✓	✓	x	✓
Confidentiality	20	✓	✓	✓	✓	✓	✓	✓
Benefits and risks of participation	20	✓	✓	✓	✓	✓	✓	✓
Limitations of risk of research on incapables	11	✓	✓	✓	x	x	x	✓
Inducement to participate	14	✓	✓	x	x	✓	x	✓
Consent of incapables	15	✓	✓	✓	x	✓	✓	✓
Research involving children	16	✓	✓	✓	x	✓	✓	✓
Ethical review of externally sponsored research	9	✓	x	x	x	x	x	✓
Information in the I.C.	11	✓	x	✓	x	x	✓	✓
Who is responsible for collecting the I.C.	8	✓	x	x	x	x	x	✓

(Continued)

Table 2.3b (Cont.)

19 Protections	Frequency of Protections	Malaysia		Nigeria	Oman	Pakistan		Qatar
		Malaysian guideline for good clinical practice	Guideline of the MMC – clinical trials and biomedical research	National code of health research ethics	Guidelines for research proposal to be submitted for review	Code of ethics for medical and dental practitioners	Ethical research committee guidelines	Guidelines, regulations, and policies for research involving human subjects
Research with limited resources	1	✗	✗	✓	✗	✗	✗	✗
Research involving vulnerable persons	13	✓	✓	✓	✗	✓	✓	✓
Compensation	12	✓	✓	✓	✗	✓	✓	✓
Strengthening ethical and scientific capacity	9	✗	✗	✓	✗	✗	✗	✓
Obligation to provide healthcare	5	✗	✗	✗	✗	✗	✗	✗
Women as research subjects	7	✗	✗	✓	✗	✗	✗	✓
Equitable distribution of burdens and benefits	6	✗	✓	✗	✓	✗	✗	✓
Total number of protections		14	12	14	5	10	9	17

Key:

✓ = Protection present

✗ = Protection absent

Different result to Alahmad et al. (2012)

Abbreviations:

I.C. = Informed consent

E.C. = Ethics committee

Table 2.3c Ethical protections stated in 24 documents of 18 OIC Countries

19 Protections	Frequency of Protections	Saudi Arabia				Sudan	Turkey	UAE	Uganda	
		SFDA clinical trial requirement guidelines	The law of ethics of research on living creatures	Implementing regulations of the law of ethics of research on living creatures	Ethics of medical profession	Guidelines for ethical conduct: Research involving human subjects	Regulation on clinical trials	Guidance for conducting clinical trials based on drugs/medicinal products and good clinical practice	National drug authority guidelines for the conduct of clinical trials	National guidelines for research involving humans as research participants
Informed consent	23	✓	✓	✓	✓	✓	✓	✓	✓	✓
E. C.	22	✓	✓	✓	✓	✓	✓	✓	✓	✓
Scientific validity	19	✓	✓	✓	✓	✓	✓	✓	✗	✓
Confidentiality	20	✓	✓	✓	✗	✓	✓	✓	✓	✓
Benefits and risks of participation	20	✓	✓	✓	✓	✓	✓	✓	✗	✓
Limitations of risk of research on incapables	11	✓	✗	✓	✗	✓	✓	✗	✗	✓

(Continued)

Table 2.3c (Cont.)

19 Protections	Frequency of Protections	Saudi Arabia				Sudan	Turkey	UAE	Uganda	
		SFDA clinical trial requirement guidelines	The law of ethics of research on living creatures	Implementing regulations of the law of ethics of research on living creatures	Ethics of medical profession	Guidelines for ethical conduct: Research involving human subjects	Regulation on clinical trials	Guidance for conducting clinical trials based on drugs/medicinal products and good clinical practice	National drug authority guidelines for the conduct of clinical trials	National guidelines for research involving humans as research participants
Inducement to participate	14	✓	✓	✓	✓	✓	✓	×	×	✓
Consent of incapables	15	✓	×	✓	×	✓	✓	×	×	✓
Research involving children	16	✓	✓	✓	×	✓	✓	×	×	✓
Ethical review of externally sponsored research	9	✓	×	✓	×	✓	×	✓	×	✓
Information in the I.C.	11	✓	×	✓	×	✓	×	✓	×	✓
Who is responsible for collecting the I.C.	8	✓	×	✓	×	✓	×	×	×	✓

Research with limited resources	1	✗	✗	✗	✗	✗	✗	✗	✗
Research involving vulnerable persons	13	✗	✓	✓	✗	✓	✓	✗	✓
Compensation	12	✓	✗	✓	✓	✓	✗	✗	✓
Strengthening ethical and scientific capacity	9	✓	✓	✓	✓	✗	✗	✗	✓
Obligation to provide healthcare	5	✓	✗	✓	✓	✗	✗	✗	✓

(Continued)

Table 2.3c (Cont.)

19 Protections	Frequency of Protections	Saudi Arabia				Sudan	Turkey	UAE	Uganda	
		SFDA clinical trial requirement guidelines	The law of ethics of research on living creatures	Implementing regulations of the law of ethics of research on living creatures	Ethics of medical profession	Guidelines for ethical conduct: Research involving human subjects	Regulation on clinical trials	Guidance for conducting clinical trials based on drugs/medicinal products and good clinical practice	National drug authority guidelines for the conduct of clinical trials	National guidelines for research involving humans as research participants
Women as research subjects	7	✗	✓	✗	✗	✓	✓	✗	✗	✓
Equitable distribution of burdens and benefits	6	✗	✗	✗	✗	✓	✗	✗	✗	✓
Total number of protections		15	10	16	6	18	11	7	3	18

Abbreviations:

I.C. = Informed consent

E.C. = Ethics committee

Key:

✓ = Protection present

✗ = Protection absent

Different result to Alahmad et al. (2012)

Table 2.4a Mention of Islam, Islamic sources or the Muslim religio-cultural context in ten documents from eight OIC countries

Country name	Kingdom of Bahrain	Bangladesh	Arab Republic of Egypt	Indonesia	Islamic Republic of Iran	Jordan	Kuwait	Lebanon
Guideline Name	Ethical guidelines for health research	National research ethics guideline	Professional ethics regulations	Indonesian health act no. 23/1992 section on health research, article 69	Protection code of the human subject in research	Law of clinical studies	Ethical guidelines for bio-medical research	Law of medical ethics
Guidelines contain reference to Islam or Islamic sources or Muslim culture	✗	✓	✓	✗	✓	✗	✗	✗
Nominal mention, i.e., in preamble only	✗	✗	✗	✗	✗	✗	✗	✗
Mention in reference to healthcare	✗	✓	✓	✗	✓	✗	✗	✗
Mention in reference to research	✗	✓	✓	✗	✓	✗	✗	✗
Role of religious leader in REC	✗	✓	✗	✗	✗	✗	✗	✗
Female consent	✗	✓	✗	✗	✗	✗	✗	✗

(Continued)

Table 2.4a (Cont.)

Country name	Kingdom of Bahrain	Bangladesh	Arab Republic of Egypt	Indonesia	Islamic Republic of Iran	Jordan	Kuwait	Lebanon
Guideline Name	Ethical guidelines for health research	National research ethics guideline	Professional ethics regulations	Indonesian health act no. 23/1992 section onhealth research, article 69	Protection code of the human subject in research	Law of clinical studies	Ethical guidelines for biomedical research	Law of medical ethics
Couple's consent for placental, foetal or umbilical cord research	✗	✓	✗	✗	✗	✗	✗	✗
Observing of religious values when conducting medical research	✗	✗	✓	✗	✓	✗	✗	✗
Care and religious considerations when conducting line-age research	✗	✗	✓	✗	✗	✗	✗	✗
Mention of Islamic principles, e.g., preservation of life	✗	✗	✗	✗	✗	✗	✗	✗
Consideration of Shariah when handling biological substances	✗	✗	✗	✗	✗	✗	✗	✗

Observance of Shariah when conducting research on aborted foetuses	x	x	x	x	x	x
Recruitment of women of child-bearing age must be reconsidered if contraception cannot be used for religious reasons	x	x	x	x	x	x
Reference to Islamic research ethics guideline, e.g., IOMS	x	x	x	x	x	x
Role of religious leaders in guideline development	x	x	x	✓	x	x

(Continued)

Table 2.4a (Cont.)

Country name	Kingdom of Bahrain	Bangladesh	Arab Republic of Egypt	Indonesia	Islamic Republic of Iran	Jordan	Kuwait	Lebanon
Guideline Name	Ethical guidelines for health research	National research ethics guideline	Professional ethics regulations	Indonesian health act no. 23/1992 section onhealth research, article 69	Protection code of the human subject in research	Law of clinical studies	Ethical guidelines for biomedical research	Law of medical ethics
Role of Islamic law in guideline development	x	x	x	x	x	x	x	x
Ethical guidance is primarily derived from God via the Qur'an and Sunnah	x	x	x	x	x	x	x	x
Medical professionals should embody Islamic virtues, e.g., perfection, sincerity	x	x	x	x	x	x	x	x
Specific references to the Qur'an	x	x	x	x	x	x	x	x
Specific references to the Hadith	x	x	x	x	x	x	x	x

Aim of researcher and research is obedience to God – intension "*Niyyah*" of researcher is key	✗	✗	✗	✗	✗	✗	✗
Gender relations, e.g., seclusion with female patients	✗	✗	✗	✗	✗	✗	✗
Aim of research must comply with *Shariah*	✗	✗	✗	✗	✗	✗	✗
Genetic research should be conducted within remit of *Shariah*	✗	✗	✗	✗	✗	✗	✗
Ensure oversight of local RECs to ensure compliance with *Shariah*	✗	✗	✗	✗	✗	✗	✗

(Continued)

Table 2.4a (Cont.)

Country name	Kingdom of Bahrain	Bangladesh	Arab Republic of Egypt	Indonesia	Islamic Republic of Iran	Jordan	Kuwait	Lebanon
Guideline Name	Ethical guidelines for health research	National research ethics guideline	Professional ethics regulations	Indonesian health act no. 23/1992 section on health research, article 69	Protection code of the human subject in research	Law of clinical studies	Ethical guidelines for biomedical research	Law of medical ethics
REC will ensure there is no violation of *Shariah* before approving research	✗	✗	✗	✗	✗	✗	✗	✗
REC will ensure human research will not cause harm, as defined by the *Shariah*, to participants	✗	✗	✗	✗	✗	✗	✗	✗
Research on cloning prohibited due to *Shariah*	✗	✗	✗	✗	✗	✗	✗	✗
Consideration of *Shariah* and opinion of religious scholar when deciding penalties for when there is violations of the law	✗	✗	✗	✗	✗	✗	✗	✗

Table 2.4b Mention of Islam, Islamic sources or the Muslim religio-cultural context in ten documents from eight OIC countries

Country name	Malaysia		Nigeria	Oman	Pakistan		Qatar	Saudi Arabia			
Guideline Name	Malaysian guideline for good clinical practice	Guideline of the MMC – Clinical trials and biomedical research	National code of health research ethics	Guidelines for research proposal to be submitted for Review	Code of ethics for medical and dental practitioners	Ethical research committee guidelines	Guidelines, regulations and policies for research involving human subjects	SFDA clinical trial requirement guidelines	The law of ethics of research on living creatures	Implementing regulations of the law of ethics of research on living creatures	Ethics of medical profession
Guidelines contain reference to Islam or Islamic sources or Muslim culture	x	x	✓	x	✓	x	✓	x	✓	✓	✓
Nominal mention, i.e., in preamble only	x	x	x	x	x	x	x	x	x	x	x
Mention in reference to healthcare	x	x	x	x	✓	x	x	x	✓	✓	✓
Mention in reference to research	x	x	✓	x	✓	x	✓	x	✓	✓	✓

(Continued)

Table 2.4b (Cont.)

Country name	Malaysia	Nigeria	Oman	Pakistan	Qatar	Saudi Arabia
Role of religious leader in REC	✗	✓	✗	✗	✓	✗
Female consent	✗	✗	✗	✗	✓	✗
Couple's consent for placental, foetal or umbilical cord research	✗	✗	✗	✗	✗	✗
Observing of religious values when conducting medical research	✗	✗	✗	✗	✗	✗
Care and religious consideration when conducting lineage research	✗	✗	✗	✗	✗	✗
Mention of Islamic principles, e.g., preservation of life	✗	✗	✗	✓	✗	✗

Consideration of *Shariah* when handling biological substances	x	x	x	x	x	x	x	x	✓	✓	x
Observance of *Shariah* when conducting research on aborted foetuses	x	x	x	x	x	x	x	x	✓	✓	x
Recruitment of women of child-bearing age must be reconsidered if contraception cannot be used for religious reasons	x	x	x	x	x	x	x	x	x	x	x
Reference to Islamic research ethics guideline, e.g., IOMS	x	x	x	x	x	x	x	x	x	x	x
Role of religious leaders in guideline development	x	x	x	x	x	x	x	x	x	x	✓

(Continued)

Table 2.4b (Cont.)

Country name	Malaysia	Nigeria	Oman	Pakistan	Qatar	Saudi Arabia		
Role of Islamic law in guideline development	✗	✗	✗	✗	✗	✗	✓	✓
Ethical guidance is primarily derived from God via the Qur'an and Sunnah	✗	✗	✗	✗	✗	✗	✗	✓
Medical professionals should embody Islamic virtues, e.g., perfection, sincerity	✗	✗	✗	✗	✗	✗	✗	✓
Specific references to the Qur'an	✗	✗	✗	✗	✗	✗	✗	✓
Specific references to the Hadith	✗	✗	✗	✗	✗	✗	✗	✓
Aim of researcher and research is obedience to God – intension "Niyyah" of	✗	✗	✗	✗	✗	✗	✗	✓

Gender relations, e.g., seclusion with female patients	x	x	x	x	x	x	x	✓
Aim of research must comply with *Shariah*	x	x	x	x	x	x	✓	✓
Genetic research should be conducted within remit of *Shariah*	x	x	x	x	x	x	✓	x
Ensure oversight of local RECs to ensure compliance with *Shariah*	x	x	x	x	x	x	✓	x
REC will ensure there is no violation of *Shariah* before approving research	x	x	x	x	x	x	✓	x

(Continued)

Table 2.4b (Cont.)

Country name	Malaysia	Nigeria	Oman	Pakistan	Qatar	Saudi Arabia			
REC will ensure human research will not cause harm, as defined by the *Shariah*, to participants	x	x	x	x	x	x	x	✓	x
Research on cloning prohibited due to *Shariah*	x	x	x	x	x	x	x	✓	x
Consideration of *Shariah* and opinion of religious scholar when deciding penalties for when there is violations of the law	x	x	x	x	x	x	x	✓	x
Total	0	3	0	4	4	0	7	18	15

Table 2.4c Mention of Islam, Islamic sources or the Muslim religio-cultural context in ten documents from eight OIC countries

Country name	Sudan	Turkey	UAE	Uganda	Uganda	Total
Guideline Name	National guidelines for ethical conduct of research involving human subjects	Regulation on clinical trials	Guidance for conducting clinical trials based on drugs/medicinal products and good clinical practice	National drug authority guidelines for the conduct of clinical trials	National guidelines for research involving humans as research participants	
Guidelines contain reference to Islam or Islamic sources or Muslim culture	✓	x	x	x	x	10
Nominal mention, i.e., in preamble only	x	x	x	x	x	0
Mention in reference to healthcare	x	x	x	x	x	7
Mention in reference to research	✓	x	x	x	x	10
Role of religious leader in REC	✓	x	x	x	x	6
Female consent	x	x	x	x	x	4
Couple's consent for placental, foetal or umbilical cord research	x	x	x	x	x	2
Observing of religious values when conducting medical research	x	x	x	x	x	5

(Continued)

Table 2.4c (Cont.)

Guideline Name	Sudan National guidelines for ethical conduct of research involving human subjects	Turkey Regulation on clinical trials	UAE Guidance for conducting clinical trials based on drugs/medicinal products and good clinical practice	Uganda National drug authority guidelines for the conduct of clinical trials	National guidelines for research involving humans as research participants	Total
Care and religious consideration when conducting lineage research	✗	✗	✗	✗	✗	2
Mention of Islamic principles, e.g., preservation of life	✗	✗	✗	✗	✗	2
Consideration of *Shariah* when handling biological substances	✗	✗	✗	✗	✗	2
Observance of *Shariah* when conducting research on aborted foetuses	✗	✗	✗	✗	✗	2
Recruitment of women of child-bearing age must be reconsidered if contraception cannot be used for religious reasons	✓	✗	✗	✗	✗	1
Reference to Islamic research ethics guideline, e.g., IOMS	✓	✗	✗	✗	✗	1
Role of religious leaders in guideline development	✗	✗	✗	✗	✗	2
Role of Islamic law in guideline development	✗	✗	✗	✗	✗	2

Ethical guidance is primarily derived from God via the Qur'an and Sunnah	x	x	x	x	1
Medical professionals should embody Islamic virtues, e.g., perfection, sincerity	x	x	x	x	1
Specific references to the Qur'an	x	x	x	x	1
Specific references to the Hadith	x	x	x	x	1
Aim of researcher and research is obedience to God – intension "Niyyah" of researcher is key	x	x	x	x	1
Gender relations, e.g., seclusion with female patients	x	x	x	x	1
Aim of research must comply with Shariah	x	x	x	x	2
Genetic research should be conducted within remit of Shariah	x	x	x	x	1

(Continued)

Table 2.4c (Cont.)

Country name	Sudan	Turkey	UAE	Uganda		Total
Guideline Name	National guidelines for ethical conduct of research involving human subjects	Regulation on clinical trials	Guidance for conducting clinical trials based on drugs/medicinal products and good clinical practice	National drug authority guidelines for the conduct of clinical trials	National guidelines for research involving humans as research participants	Total
Ensure oversight of local RECs to ensure compliance with *Shariah*	x				x	1
REC will ensure there is no violation of *Shariah* before approving research	x				x	1
REC will ensure human research will not cause harm, as defined by the *Shariah*, to participants	x				x	1
Research on cloning prohibited due to *Shariah*	x				x	1
Consideration of *Shariah* and opinion of religious scholar when deciding penalties for when there is violations of the law	x				x	1
Total	5	0	0	0	0	

In addition to the variation in the presence of guidelines, there is also marked variation in the level of protections offered. For example, the guidelines from Qatar mention extensively the protections highlighted by the international guidelines used as a reference in this study. This may be because Qatar has more recently established itself as a research hub and so has been able to learn from its neighbours about the ethical requirements for international research and publication.

Informed consent and the need for ethics review do feature heavily within the guidelines, however, very few mention the obligation for providing healthcare. Although healthcare is free for nationals in countries like the UAE, Qatar and Saudi Arabia, migrant workers and expatriates are not offered free service. An obligation to provide healthcare for these groups may need to be specifically cited in such guidelines.

Overall, the majority of the countries within the OIC have either no guidelines or documentation with major deficiencies. This is a cause for concern, as it is likely that such absences will affect human subject research in these places and may even attract industry and research intuitions to carry out research without the necessary concern for essential protections (Kermani, 2010). It may be that countries without specific guidelines or those with a paucity of protections may simply be employing international guidelines like CIOMS. However, only one example of this was found, which was from the Universiti Brunei Darussalam (please see Table 3.2 for details of correspondence), which specifies use of WHO guidelines. Further research is necessary to comprehensively document the nature and extent of ethical guidelines and protections within the OIC.

Presence of guidelines and levels of protections mentioned do not equate to ethical research

Although this review has emphasised the search and analysis of guidelines within the OIC countries, it is important to highlight here that although 21 countries do have guidelines, some of which that are extensively detailed, it does not indicate that research in these countries is being conducted ethically. Neither does it prove that those with more extensive guidelines are likely to have fewer breaches of ethical codes than those with limited or no guidelines. What would be required is a collaborative effort for an extensive piece of empirical research to look in detail at how research is conducted within the OIC, what ethical protections are implemented and what governance processes exist to address breaches in ethical conduct. There is also a need for collaborative efforts to equip those countries without guidelines or ethical expertise with the means to prevent exploitation and ensure ethical research.

Reference to Islam, Islamic sources and the Muslim context

Eight of the 18 countries that have guidelines mention Islam, Islamic sources and/or the Muslim context. All of the documents that have a mention of the faith do so beyond a nominal mention. Alahmad et al. (2012) suggested that the guidelines they studied did not mention any references or codes from Islamic medical entities. However, this study shows that the guidelines reviewed do, in some instances, make extensive consideration of an Islamic perspective and/or a Muslim context, including issues around research on women, which Alahmad et al. (2012) previously mentioned were absent from the guidelines they had reviewed.

A concurrent review of the literature helps to shed further light on how the role of Islam is manifest within biomedical research practice. In Iran, for example, a medical ethics research centre was established in 1993, and the National Committee for Medical Research was founded in 1998. The committee has the following responsibilities: "To apply Islamic, legal and moral principles to biomedical research; To guard human rights and legally protect the participants, the researchers and the institutes involved in research; To promote mandatory inclusion of advisors on ethical issues in all research projects at universities, private research foundations and industries" (Larijani et al., 2005, p. 1064).

The National Committee has also helped establish regional committees for reviewing ethical issues that arise from medical research. Iran now has regional committees in over 40 medical universities throughout the country. In 2000, the Ministry of Health and Medical Education prepared a guideline comprising 26 National Codes of Ethics for biomedical researchers. It was prepared in accordance with CIOMS and the Helsinki Declaration. Further, the authors state that the codes have been customized according to the *Shi'a* tradition, which is the official religion of Iran (Larijani et al., 2005).

Larijani et al further mention that:

> In the Islamic Republic of Iran, ethical issues are discussed among physicians, legal experts and religious scholars. The principles of bioethics and solutions to ethical problems are therefore derived from the Islamic legal rulings. They are updated in the light of the Holy Quran, the traditions of the Prophet of Islam (Peace Be Upon Him), the consensus of scholars, and human wisdom or intellect.
>
> (Larijani et al., 2005, p. 1063)

An examination of the Iranian 26 national codes of ethics for biomedical research reveals that they do not explicitly mention Islamic sources, reference God or detail which parts of the codes may have been derived directly from the *Shi'a* tradition. However, the authors discuss that a rigorous consultation between Islamic scholars and biomedical experts took place in order to construct the codes. This suggests that, although the wording may be the same for both secular and Islamic guidelines, the consultation process involving Islamic scholars may be valuable, both for the acceptance and applicability of the guidelines, as well as wider education and awareness.

The guideline search and review highlights that consultation with researchers, scholars and physicians is key in order to understand the process by which, in countries like Iran, ethical questions pertaining to research are chosen, prioritised and addressed through a process of communal enquiry. Little work has been done to investigate empirically the dynamics of meetings comprised of scholars of religious texts and professionals in the clinical/research context. Chapters 3 through 6 provide more details of such encounters in biomedical research ethics deliberations in Iran and Malaysia.

Other guidelines, such as the Saudi Arabia research ethics guidelines, state the importance of the character of a medical doctor and/or researcher, emphasizing virtues such as "honesty", "piety" and "sincerity".[11] These are not simply mentioned as virtues of a clinician/researcher but of a Muslim practicing his profession, with key references to the *Qur'an* and the example of the Prophet Muhammad. Furthermore, the review in this chapter shows that in Saudi Arabia, Islamic opinion is sought on what research can be done, for example, exploring the permissibility of stem cell research, genetic manipulation or use of biobanks, as well as how clinical research should be conducted, with an Islamic scholar being appointed on each ethics committee and being involved in the penalization process when breaches in protocol occur (see Table 2.4).

Women in research

Following a review of the literature, a key theme identified in relation to Islam and biomedical research ethics was the role and involvement of women in research (Suleman, 2016). In particular, the review highlighted how the status of women is a commonly disputed topic within Islam. Although spiritually equal to men, where the *Qur'an* emphasises this spiritual equality, (*The* Holy Qur'an, Chapter 16, verse 97), physically, women are offered the protection of men through their fathers, guardians or husbands (*The* Holy Qur'an, Chapter 4, verse 34). This *Quranic* principle is taken to imply that women are more vulnerable and, therefore, need protection. The application of the latter principle often leads to discordance within the Muslim community. For example, within research, some authors suggest that a married woman may only participate if she has first sought the permission of her husband (Afifi, 2007). A husband may not, however, force his wife to participate in a trial (Afifi, 2007). Seeing it as a religious duty, women may consider their husband's permission as imperative, and such a decision may be described as her exercising her second order autonomy (Keyserlingk, 1993). Others have argued, however, that it is not in accordance with a woman's human rights to have to seek her husband's permission before participating in a trial (Fadel, 2010)(see IOMS guidelines below).

Another important ethical consideration is that women are often marginalised in communities and do not have access to healthcare. Does such a religious position empower women to have the necessary discussions with the male members of the household, where such conversations may be necessary and

11 Saudi Council for Health Specialists. (2014). Ethics of the medical profession. http:// dent.ksu.edu.sa/sites/default/files/rr/35.pdf (Last accessed June 2014).

common, or does it cause them to withdraw further from accessing services? The ambiguity in the interpretation of the normative texts, however, reveals that more may be at play in determining the gender roles in Muslim communities. It would require an empirical investigation to explore communities where women are required to seek permission and whether the religious texts influence these social norms or cultural traditions shared by other faith communities in the region, and they are, therefore, independent of religion. Such an empirical analysis involving the role of women in research in Malaysia and Iran is presented in Chapter 5.

Given such findings from the literature review, it was deemed pertinent to further analyse research ethics guidelines to evaluate the role of women in research. Four of the guidelines reviewed have clauses specifically mentioning the enrolment and role of women in research. The Bangladesh guidelines state that: "The mother's decision to donate foetal tissue is sufficient for the use of the tissue unless the father objects in writing", and the use of stem cells requires "free and informed consent from both of the parents of the newborn. If there is disagreement between parents, the umbilical cord and placenta cannot be used for research".[12]

In the Saudi Arabian guideline, "Ethics of the medical profession",[13] there is reference to a *fatwah* (legal edict), which states that a woman is free to consent to treatment unless it involves procedures "relating to reproduction, such as usage of contraceptives, or hysterectomy or any other procedure specifically those leading to infertility." The *fatwah* referenced is from the "Decision of the Supreme Council of Ulama Decision No: 173". Although this is mentioned in reference to healthcare, it may also apply to clinical research. The other Saudi Arabian guideline, "The law of ethics of research on living creatures",[14] mentions that a researcher may not initiate research on a pregnant woman unless the informed consent of both the pregnant woman and her husband is obtained.

The Qatar guideline states:

> If the research holds out the prospect of direct benefit solely to the foetus, then the consent of the pregnant woman and the father is obtained in accord with the informed consent provisions described above except that the father's consent need not be obtained if he is unable to consent because of

12 Medical Research Council (Bangladesh). (2013). National research ethics guideline. http://www.bgmc.edu.bd/ethics_ex.php?arid=19 (Last accessed 20 March 2014). Guideline can be obtained from info@bmrcbd.

13 Saudi Council for Health Specialists. (2014). Ethics of the medical profession. http://dent.ksu.edu.sa/sites/default/files/rr/35.pdf (Last accessed June 2014).

14 Law of ethics of research on living creatures. Issued under Royal decree no. M/59 dated 14.9.1431 AH, Ministerial resolution no. 321 dated 13.9.1431 AH and Circular of the Minister of Justice no. 13/T/4202 dated 3.4.1432 AH. (2014). http://old.sfda.gov.sa/NR/rdonlyres/D6892236-AF58-41B2-9AC4-DE0E3BF53380/0/ClinicalTrialsRequirmentsGuidelines_12.pdf (Last accessed June 2014).

unavailability, incompetence, or temporary incapacity or the pregnancy resulted from rape or incest.[15]

Although the Qatari and Bangladeshi guidelines do not reference Islam as the source for the reasoning behind the need for the husband's consent, they do require further analysis. The Saudi Arabian guideline that cites a religious edict or *fatwah* highlights the role of religious authority in formulating healthcare and research policies. It may be important to consider the religio-cultural necessity of applying such religious dicta within research. Although *fatawah* or scholarly opinions are formulated to enrich the law, there is scope for differences of opinions between scholars, and a scholar him/herself may change an opinion over time. The findings here suggest that more work needs to be done to assess the role of *fatawah* in biomedical research.

IOMS: The international ethical guidelines for biomedical research involving human subjects "An Islamic perspective"

An adaptation of the international guideline CIOMS, which has been produced for use within the Muslim world, was published by IOMS in 2005 (IOMS, 2005, pp. 121–276). The IOMS guideline reviews the CIOMS publication clause by clause, offering an Islamic perspective on the entire guideline. However, it is unclear from the IOMS guideline and related publications (Fadel, 2010) what method was employed for the production of the so-called "Islamic perspectives" on, for example, the enrolment of women in research. Although the IOMS guideline states that a woman's individual consent should be sought, it also offers that, although not a requirement, "it is preferable to obtain the husband's consent" (IOMS, 2005, p. 233). The latter is ambiguous, however, with no details about which circumstances would necessitate a husband's opinion. It would be useful, therefore, to know empirically how Muslims researchers, who use IOMS or other such resources as a guide, implement this clause.

In summary, there have been attempts in some countries to develop guidelines that take into consideration the Islamic normative sources and local Muslim contexts. The extent to which such consideration is made and how considerations are reflected in the deliberations and authorship of the guidelines varies. Countries like Saudi Arabia and Iran describe extensive involvement of religious scholars in the guideline development process. The international IOMS (2005) guideline that was produced in collaboration with numerous scholars and biomedical experts is the first attempt to author a transnational research ethics guideline that incorporates Islamic perspectives. It is, however, difficult to determine from purely a textual analysis to what extent these guidelines offer cosmetic or substantive Islamic ethical perspectives. In order to more fully determine the extent to which these

15 Qatar Supreme Council of Health. (2009). Guidelines, regulations and policies for research involving human subjects. http://qatar-weill.cornell.edu/research/pdf/Minis try%20Guidelines.doc (Last accessed June 2014).

guidelines offer an Islamic ethical framework for the biomedical research context, the textual content of these guidelines would have to be analysed alongside their contextual application, through an empirical study of how researchers and research ethics committees employ their content.

Conclusion

This chapter presented a review of the current international, national and institutional ethical guidelines found within the OIC. Although attempts have been made by some countries to offer protections comparable to international standards, most of the countries do not have guidelines, or they have documents with major deficiencies. Another important consideration highlighted by this review is the role of Islam, its sources and the Muslim context within the research ethics discourse. However, in many of the guidelines, the methods employed to offer an Islamic perspective and how these perspectives ought to be incorporated in the work of biomedical researchers is unclear. Although the application of Islamic principles is varied and inconsistent, the review emphasises the role of religion and religious authority in underlining research priorities, guidelines and conduct, which requires further study to ascertain its impact on ethical decision-making.

Both the literature (Suleman, 2016) and guideline review reveal that an exploration of Islam's influence on research ethics and the role of religious scholars and normative Islamic sources in the construction of guidelines or within research ethics decision-making is an area that is understudied and requires further research. This textual study is complemented by an empirical analysis to investigate if and how Islam influences the ethical decision-making of researchers, REC members, guideline developers and Islamic scholars in the biomedical research context through fieldwork in two case study sites, Malaysia and Iran. These sites were chosen due to their extensive involvement in research, prevalence of research ethics guidelines and RECs as well as their deep socio-political commitment to Islam.

The empirical study required the construction of an interview guide and analytical frame (Chapter 8). The themes found within the literature and guideline review pertinent to the question of Islam's influence on biomedical research ethics, such as the role of scholars or the personal characteristics of the physician/researcher, were used to inform the development of the research tools for the empirical study. Chapters 3 through 6 will detail findings from interviews conducted in the two countries and illuminate how Islam plays a role in biomedical research ethics decision-making.

Bibliography

Afifi, R. Y. (2007). Biomedical research ethics: An Islamic view part II. *International Journal of Surgery*, 5(6), 381–383.
Alahmad, G., Al-Jumah, M. & Dierickx, K. (2012). Review of national research ethics regulations and guidelines in middle eastern Arab countries. *BMC Medical Ethics*, 13(1), doi:10.1186/1472-6939-13-34.

CIOMS. (2002). International ethical guidelines for biomedical research involving human subjects. www.fhi360.org/training/fr/retc/pdf_files/cioms.pdf (Last accessed 15 January 2020).

Fadel, H. E. (2010). Ethics of clinical research: An Islamic perspective. *Journal of the Islamic Medical Association of North America*, 42(2).

IOMS (Islamic Organization for Medical Sciences). (2004). International Conference on "Islamic Code of Medical Ethics". http://islamset.net/ioms/code2004/index.html (Last accessed 15 January 2020).

IOMS (Islamic Organization for Medical Sciences). (2005). International ethical guidelines for biomedical research involving human subjects "an Islamic perspective". In A. R. El-Gendy & A. R. A. Al-Awadi, (Eds.). *The international Islamic code for medical and health ethics.* (Vol. 2, 121–276). Kuwait: Islamic Organization for Medical Sciences.

Kermani, F. (2010). How to run clinical trials in the Middle East. *SCRIP*(February), 1–8.

Keyserlingk, E. W. (1993). Ethics codes and guidelines for health care and research: can respect for autonomy be a multi-cultural principle. In J. R. Coombs & E. Winkler (Eds.). *Applied ethics: A reader* (pp. 319–415). Oxford: Blackwell Publishers.

Larijani, B., Zahedi, F. & Malek-Afzali, H. (2005). Medical ethics in the Islamic Republic of Iran. *East Mediterr Health J*, 11(5–6), 1061–1072.

Sachedina, A. (2009). *Islamic biomedical ethics: Principles and application.* New York: Oxford University Press.

Silverman, H. (Ed.). (2017). *Research ethics in the Arab region.* Cham, Switzerland: Springer International Publishing.

Suleman, M. (2016). Contributions and ambiguities in Islamic research ethics and research conducted in Muslim contexts: I – A thematic review of the literature. *Journal of Health and Culture*, 1(1): 46–57.

Suleman, M. (2017). Biomedical research ethics in the Islamic context. Reflections on and challenges for Islamic Bioethics. In A. Bagheri & K. A. Ali (Eds.). *Islamic bioethics: Current issues and challenges* (Vol. 2, 197–228). (Singapore: World Scientific.

The Holy Qur'an. Chapter 4, verse 34. http://corpus.quran.com/translation.jsp?chapter=4&verse=34 (Last accessed 2 March 2016).

The Holy Qur'an. Chapter 16, verse 97. http://corpus.quran.com/translation.jsp?chapter=16&verse=97 (Last accessed 27 January 2014).

WHO (World Health Organisation). (2005). Islamic code of medical and health ethics. http://applications.emro.who.int/docs/EM_RC52_7_en.pdf (Last accessed 20 March 2014).

3 Role of institutional forms of Islam in biomedical research ethics

Religious texts, scholars and their legal edicts

One of the most important themes arising from my analysis of the interview transcripts and reviews of detailed field notes was the significant influence of the institutional forms of Islam within the context of biomedical research in Malaysia and Iran. My analysis of the data presented here will show how Islam influences ethical decision-making within biomedical research today through religious texts, scholars and their legal edicts, why these sources have come to be recognised as the "Islamic authority" and how this authority is evolving. The purpose of this chapter is to outline how these different structures interact and present themselves in the context of biomedical research and to lay the foundations for the more substantive discussions on specific ethical issues arising from the enrolment of women into studies and HIV research, which will be covered in subsequent chapters.

In order to explore how Islam and the Muslim context affect ethical decision-making within biomedical research, participants were asked about how such issues were raised and why and what processes were implemented to address them. The role and function of RECs in Malaysia has been understudied (Yusuf, 2014), and, prior to this study, the influence of Islam and the Muslim context within their remit has not been investigated. Although more work has been done to review and explain the role of Islam within guideline development in Iran, very little is known about the types of issues that require consideration from an Islamic perspective and how these are dealt with in the context of biomedical research.

This chapter, where relevant, also presents a comparison of the views expressed in Iran and Malaysia and attempts to explain where differences occur and why. The aim, however, is not to provide a direct comparison of the views and experiences in both countries. It is to present the broader differences that are appreciable from the views of participants to try and explain these differences based on the religious and geopolitical contexts of the two countries.[1]

---

1 For a detailed account of study site selection and a brief background on Malaysia and Iran, please see Chapter 8.

The role of Islam and its normative sources in how ethical issues are identified and raised by RECs and researchers

In both settings, issues emerging from biomedical research proposals and methods that may carry religious concerns are raised at multiple levels. In Malaysia these include the institutional review boards (IRBs) and/or the Malaysian Medical Council (MMC)[2] as well as the National Committee for Clinical Research (NCCR). In Iran these include the institutional RECs, the national Medical Ethics and Medical History Research Centre (MEHRC), the Ministry of Health and Medical Education (MOHME) as well as the parliament and Guardian Council. In both countries consideration at the individual clinician/research level through personal experience and/or education and training plays an important role in the identification of ethical issues that may then require deliberation from an Islamic perspective.

Islamic ethico-legal issues emerging from personal experience

Many of the participants, as REC members, guideline developers, or researchers, expressed how their own experiences and ethical considerations informed their decisions about what they considered morally problematic and how they then went about addressing such issues. One researcher described how his personal deliberations as a researcher and REC member involved considerations of Islamic perspectives and the Muslim context within which he works:

> For example, those researches around sexual health – going inside the private structure of their lives – to ask about sexual behaviours. For example, a research ethics committee must be or should be more sensitive about these things when you go and knock on the house door and ask people about these. It is dangerous in some parts of the country to ask those questions, because people feel offended, feel disturbed. Then if you want respect, human dignity, you should try to educate, for example, the researchers about these things.
> (Iran Interview 1, Researcher, REC member)

Many participants in both countries expressed similar views regarding consideration of Islamic ethico-legal concerns around sensitive issues, such as sexuality, and whether and how these ought to be researched. Such views and concerns will be discussed in more detail in subsequent chapters.

Islamic ethico-legal issues emerging from RECs and national councils

Participants in both countries explained that religious issues may be flagged from the individual researcher to the level of the national ethics committee.

---

2   Malaysian Medical Council. (2020). Laws & regulations. http://www.mmc.gov.my/laws-regulations (Last accessed 24 March 2020).

Given its multi-ethnic and multicultural make-up, participants in Malaysia explained how RECs are commonly comprised of Malay, Chinese and Indian members representing many faiths, including Islam, Buddhism, Christianity, Hinduism, and no faith. Many participants also explained how the awareness and flagging of issues relating to Islam is not within the purview of only Muslim researchers and REC members; rather, those who are not Muslim describe being broadly familiar with the practices and requirements of Islam due to Malaysia's multicultural make-up:

> Religion wise, I think we understand the others well in this country. When we carry out, or in the proposal, most of the time that has been looked into by the supervisor. As I said, because we grow up in the country with different kind of ethnicity, we are so used to the background of our friends in the other religions. We know, for example, when we have animal studies we will use guinea pigs, we will not use dogs, or pigs, that kind of thing. That has been understood. We will never use that as our samples, and hence that issue doesn't arise.
>
> (Malaysia Interview 15, Researcher)

The participants in Malaysia raised an important issue in relation to preparing adequately for their study population and being respectful of their religious beliefs. Many explained how they were well versed about the impermissibility of the use of, for example, alcohol or porcine products, according to Islamic law, so either personally or at the REC level they would ensure that such materials are not included in the research intervention.

In Iran, as alcohol is banned, the potential use of alcohol-based products as research interventions was not a concern. However, researching behaviours that infringe the Islamic state law, for example, researching the consumption of alcohol or extramarital relationships, raised ethical concerns in Iran, including the safety of participants and the acceptability of researching unlawful behaviour. Here it is important to mention that in Iran, at the level of RECs, issues relating to Islamic law and those that arise from the interpretation of Islam's normative sources are considered very important. For example, one participant in Iran explained how research proposals that involved the translation of questionnaires developed in a different religio-cultural context raised issues within their REC:

> I think that their religious concern is under the umbrella of ethical codes. Many ethical codes accept these concerns and warn about these concerns, and researchers should consider these aspects of participants, religious concerns ... For example, "Have you had any experience, sexual experience, before? Do you have a sexual partner? How many partners do you have?" It's a really bad question, here in Iran, okay. You cannot ask, even from an adult, you cannot ask, "How many partners do you have?" It is not a usual question here, okay.
>
> (Iran Interview 14, Researcher, REC member)

Her experience highlights that there are specific issues that are considered particularly sensitive that relate to the religious and/or cultural context of Iran. Chapter 4 provides a deeper exploration of what these issues are and the underlying Islamic normative basis for concerns around sexual promiscuity.

Ethical concerns that require consideration from an Islamic/Muslim perspective therefore arise in many ways. Some appear through personal experience, as is seen in many other contexts globally, however, there are others that arise more formally through RECs and ministries themselves flagging issues that are considered to be religio-culturally sensitive. It is important to mention here that, unlike Malaysia, Iran also has the added nationalised layers of the Guardian Council, the Parliament and the Supreme Leader – these are authorities that ensure "Islam" is prioritised and protected in a more overt way than that seen in Malaysia. As such, a key finding here is that, in Iran, the consideration of Islamic issues that emerge within biomedical research is more centrally considered due to the country's political make-up. In Malaysia, by contrast, this happens in a more bottom-up or ad-hoc basis, relying on the experience of researchers and RECs. The way these issues are addressed is also different in the two countries. In Iran the role of Islam's normative sources and Islamic scholars is more centrally established, whereas in Malaysia this occurs within a parallel legal system of *Shariah* courts and *fatawah*. How issues are addressed and the exploration of the centralised nature of Islam's influence in Iran and the parallel nature in Malaysia will now be discussed.

The role of Islam and its normative sources in how ethical issues are addressed once identified by RECs and researchers

When issues are raised these are then discussed at multiple levels including by researchers themselves, by members of institutional RECs and/or the National/state level *fatwah* councils and/or an individually consulted mufti. In Iran there is additional potential consultation with the national MEHRC, the MOHME or the guardian council and parliament. Islam's institutional elements that are employed to address ethical issues that are identified as requiring an "Islamic" response include, traditional scholars versed in the Islamic normative sources and their interpretation, the *Shariah* or Islamic law, as well as *fatawah* or legal edicts from individual scholars or a committee of scholars.

Role of traditional scholars and the emerging role for contextual and bridge scholars

Role of scholars in RECs and national committees

The data analysis shows that there is a commitment to involve religious scholars within RECs and national prioritisation decisions in Iran, whereas in Malaysia their involvement depends on flagging of issues by researchers and/or RECs. Very few ethics committees in Malaysia have a regular Islamic scholar as a member. Participants in Iran, by contrast, explained how the membership of a Muslim scholar is integral in many RECs. In the city of Isfahan, which has been reported by some authors as being a religiously conservative part of Iran (Aghajanian & Merhyar, 1999), respondents explained how there is a commitment to developing an Islamic approach to emerging issues involving professionals and scholars. Another participant in Iran spoke about how the role and responsibility of Islamic scholars has evolved since the Revolution:

> The third issue regarding the interpretation of Islam that we have now in Iran is that the responsibility of religious government for justifying for governing the society ... before having an Islamic government that claims all of my, for example, recommendations and laws are compatible with Islam. Before that, the Principle of *Maslaha* or this public good was less noticed by *Shiite* jurists, because the government was responsible for providing public good. The king or kings were the responsible person. [The] religious sector, as a conservative sector, maybe is not in favour of doing, going and putting itself in trouble and enter[ing] issues. The easiest way is to say no ... At the same time I think the Islamic government was an opportunity [for] *Shiite* jurisprudence to say that, yes, it is possible to have such interpretation of Islam that says, for example, you can use gametes to fertilise, normal that of the gametes are not working, because [if] you have an infertility rate about 15–20%, then you should respond. Otherwise, they will go to London for doing IVF.
>
> (Iran Interview 1, Researcher, REC member)

The participant highlights a key shift in the role of religious scholars and seminaries in Iran after the establishment of the Islamic state. Once recognised as an authority, *Shi'i* scholars took on the role of responding to the Iranian society's emerging problems, and, in a way, that was more permissive than previously seen due to their newly found responsibility of ensuring "public good".

Another participant in Iran, however, explained that in her experience the involvement of a scholar within the REC was unhelpful, as he disagreed with a research proposal that involved yoga as an intervention for postpartum depression. She explained that he was unaware of the existing literature on the potential benefits of the intervention and instead suggested that the intervention ought to include recitation of the *Qur'an*. She suggested that the REC ought to reconsider the type of "scholar" that is included on the committee:

> We have a religious man, one Rouhani, in our team, but unfortunately, in my idea, his idea is not very benefi[cial] for us – our decision-making – because his idea is just only from [a] different [point] of view about this one matter. He doesn't have any information about the medicine. His knowledge is just only about the faith and the religion ... In my idea, if the committee selects some people that know faith and spirituality in the medicine, but they are practicing medicine, [then they] are more knowledgeable to the medical standard than just only [the] religious, such as [a] cleric, such as a Rouhani and something else ... in my idea, it is not useful.
>
> (Iran Interview 4, Researcher, REC member)

A bridge scholar (definition and role will be explained below) in Malaysia explained that, though not formally institutionalised, there is a growing role for religion within the bioethics discourse in Malaysia, not just from the Islamic perspective, but for all faiths:

> I think what we are seeing is that participation of religious scholars in these committees [is] being acknowledged. Not all ethics committee actually have members of the religious ... [they] do not actually have members from the religious background in the committee. Even if they are, [there are] not that many. But, like I said, the trend ... we are seeing that it is growing, not only from the Islamic perspective, actually. There are committees that actually do engage other faiths as well. As you are well aware, Malaysia is made up of people of various faiths. Like organ donation, the Ministry of Health actually engages all the various faiths to get them on board, to get their views if there are any concerns that should be known by the ministry. I think this is helpful, because it's in a form of a meaningful dialogue.
>
> One thing that I can say is that the medical fraternity seems to be acknowledging the role of religion when it comes to applying new techniques, new treatments and new medicines. I see this now being spilled over into other fields by technology. Malaysia has a committee called the Genetic Modification Advisory Council. Everything that wants to be ... everything that is being researched on regarding genetic modification has to go through this council. Currently, the council is made up of scientists, lawyers, policy makers, but they've been talking about involving religious scholars as well. If that happens, and when that happens, then definitely there is a step for it.
>
> (Malaysia Interview 32, "bridge" scholar, REC member)

When asked whether the role and input of scholars has changed in recent decades, most participants in both countries describe it as their input being more permissive and supportive of emerging research and technologies:

> I think compared to ten years ago, no. They're more open ... For example, stem cells, stem cells is the thing. Ten years ago they were quite reluctant to get involved in stem cell research, but now, after clearer discussions with scholars, we know that we cannot run away from the role of stem cells. That has shaped the interest of everybody to come and do stem cell research. The only issue is involved with commercialisation or not.
>
> (Malaysia Interview 11, Researcher, REC member)

The participant explained that the involvement of scholars, by informing and educating them about the potential uses of research outputs such as stem cells, has caused them to engage with the moral implications of such interventions and has, in fact, led to positive responses. Islamic scholarly involvement in the stem cell discussion has meant that Muslim researchers in Malaysia, who had previously been apprehensive to engage in such research, as they were unable to morally reconcile the questions posed by the technology, were provided with religious reassurance by the scholarly endorsement.

In Malaysia, given the lack of a nationalised view on "what Islam says", an important ethical consideration is the role of REC members in raising religio-ethical issues, and how these may simply reflect their own personal beliefs. RECs must be wary, therefore, of their potential normative influence:

> I think it is quite against what I believe, because I believe that we need to have a, what do you call, men and women need to be in an official marriage by … I don't know how to … The relationship must be official, and then only they can have sex or whatever. But, if you say it is before that they do it, they did that, so to me it is against the religion, first of all. If I really want to understand the issue, I will conduct research to understand the issue. Not really … how do I say this? In Malaysia, for example, the numbers of teenage pregnanc[ies] can be skyrocketing. There is an increase every year, and then a lot of babies have been thrown away in the dustbin and everywhere. If I really want to understand the issue, my aim is to help to reduce the numbers and also to reduce numbers of babies that have been thrown away. My aim is that. Not really whether they wear protection. It is not that. If I ask them whether they wear protection, and then [say], "Oh, you should wear protection", meaning that I agree that you can have sex before marriage, but you need to wear protection. Something like that. It is against my belief so if … For me you cannot do it until you get married. Then, only, I can ask whether you wear protection or not. Something like that. The discussion is on the beha-viour, and how we are going to prevent it, not really how are you going to do it without getting pregnant.
>
> (Malaysia Interview 12, Researcher, REC member)

The REC member explained how he had refused on multiple occasions to approve research that involved studying the efficacy of barrier contraception on the transmission of STIs (sexually transmitted diseases) amongst young people and sex workers. This was because he considered extramarital relationships to be against his own religious views, and that approving such studies would be sym-bolic of such activities being acceptable in wider society. How personal faith influences decisions within the biomedical research context will be explored in more detail in Chapter 6, however, here it is important to consider such experi-ences, as it highlights a particular role that Islamic scholars and the National *Fatwah* Council in Malaysia undertake. For example, a REC member explained that one of the ways to address religio-ethical concerns raised by individuals is to refer the matter up to the National *Fatwah* Council. He explained that if, espe-cially, a senior member of the REC raises a religious issue, then it was difficult for the committee to ignore. They would, therefore, refer the issue up to the National *Fatwah* Council. He found that the council may be more permissive in terms of research than individual REC members:

I think the only conflict is really due to personal convictions or personal religious convictions. Whereas, I think whenever we had to refer to the council, I found that the council tends to be a little bit less restrictive but more to do with benefits towards health, research or mankind. When we had to refer, as long as it was to benefit another person, or to benefit ... I find that the council tends to be a little bit more lax and less restrictive.

(Malaysia Interview 17, Researcher, REC member)

Community engagement role of scholars

Scholars have also been described as having a pastoral role in the ethics committees to emphasise the safety and interests of participants and in the community by being better informed of the views of the people. For example, when asked why scholars may be present in RECs or are consulted, one participant explained:

In this setup, for example, it's not the scientific research itself where there's a need for scholarly input, it's the convincing the community itself on this particular research. I think more of a social behavioural function of this scholar, rather than the input to the scientific process itself ... I think [of] their role because ... I believe still in the social/behavioural impact [of] this scholar towards the study. They should be supporting, understanding the research that is being done, and their role in supporting ... their duty will have an impact on the intervention. Not scientifically, but on the implementation in the society. I believe that is their role.

(Malaysia Interview 11, Researcher, REC member)

Role of scholars in the authorship of national guidelines

In Iran participants explained the importance of involving Islamic scholars in the drafting of national biomedical research ethics guidelines. Some authors have described the method through which Islamic values are considered within the context of bioethics in Iran:

In the Islamic Republic of Iran, ethical issues are discussed among physicians, legal experts and religious scholars. The principles of bioethics and solutions to ethical problems are therefore derived from the Islamic legal rulings. They are updated in the light of the Holy Quran, the traditions of the Prophet of Islam (Peace Be Upon Him), the consensus of scholars, and human wisdom or intellect.

(Larijani et al., 2005, p. 1063)

A key aim of this research and, in particular, the fieldwork in Iran was to analyse the process of textual and contextual consultation with religious scholars as well as reviewing how the resulting guidelines then impact practice at the individual researcher level.

One senior researcher in Iran explained that in his experience the involvement of Islamic scholars in the authorship of national research ethics guidelines was integral to the development of religio-culturally appropriate guidelines. For the authorship of the national guidelines in biomedical research ethics, there was involvement from four Islamic scholars. Members, such as clinicians and researchers, who were not formally trained scholars, also raised issues that were considered pertinent to the Islamic faith. He explained how the issue of women's involvement in research was raised during the consultation and considered distinctly by the different members:

> Among the members [with] which we were working on this project and [the] four independent religious counsellors which we had for this project, it was pretty apparent to us that it's hard to get a consensus from the group, because we had people who believed that if a female Muslim would like to participate in a clinical research, she has to ask her husband to sign the informed consent form. We had lots of discussion, and the conclusion to me was pretty interesting. It was pretty good to what the spirit of religion would agree.
>
> (Iran Interview 15, national bioethics guideline developer)

He explained how the flagging of the issue of women's enrolment in research led to disagreement amongst members, and the Islamic scholars played a key role in evaluating the issue. This consultation of scholars and researchers on the issue of female consent during the development of the national guidelines in Iran will be further analysed in Chapter 5.

The participant also explained that the involvement of scholars was to ensure the acceptance of the policy both within the national political institutions and the wider public:

> Working in a religious country, you can't ignore that very important discipline, I would say. You can't, in a religious country, you can't work on national ethical codes and ignore [the] Islamic perspective, which would be presented by an Islamic scholar. Even for full consultation workshops, for those two workshops, we invited more religious scholars ... to see how they would agree or disagree with the draft which we prepared as national ethical codes. It's a part of the discussion. You can't ignore it. You can't exclude that from the discussion. That's why we had that on board from the beginning, and otherwise, I can't see the possibility of approving those 26 codes. It's not just because it was on research ethics. In any medical ethical issues [on] which we work, I can't see the possibility of, let's say, social acceptance of those products or polic[ies] without including [the] religious perspective when you are working in a religious country like Iran.
>
> (Iran Interview 15, national bioethics guideline developer)

Another participant in Iran explained, off-the-record, that the involvement of scholars within deliberations relating to the development of guidelines is political.

She emphasised that the traditional scholars did not contribute to the discussions per se, but they were included to simply "authorise" the proceedings. She explained that scholars have to be involved in guideline development to prevent their group being accused of secularisation or changing the culture. She wanted to speak off-the-record as the role of traditional scholars in influencing guidelines and policy is a politically sensitive issue, and she did not want her views recorded and quoted directly for fear that they may be linked to her or her organisation.

In Iran it was evident from some of the participants' views and experiences that Islamic scholars play a key role in determining the "Islamic" view that is embedded into guidelines, and subsequently they ensure the acceptance of the policy both within the national political institutions and also the wider public.

In Malaysia, by contrast, Muslim scholars may be involved in guideline development; however, this process is not institutionalised or systematically driven by national policies. Such a consultation may occur in Malaysia on an ad hoc basis depending on the guidance being produced. However, during my fieldwork and interviews with institutional REC members or members of the MMC, there was no expression or consideration of formally involving Islamic scholars in the development of research ethics guidelines. Again, this may be due to Malaysia's multi-cultural and multi-ethnic make up, their commitment to ensuring the guidelines align with international standards to attract overseas research projects, or the fact that the guideline developers feel adequately equipped to ensure that the guidelines are contextually appropriate.

Bridge scholars in Malaysia – an emerging role in Islamic bioethics and an evolving tension in Islamic authority

An emerging theme from the data analysis of the interviews in Malaysia was the role of so-called "bridge scholars". One of the participants explained how he became involved in the Islamic bioethics discourse in Malaysia and is now an expert bridge scholar – one who is trained in the physical sciences but has also received a formal education in the Islamic sciences:

I've been involved with this since the late 90s. Back then, when I started, people [were] still asking "What is ethics?", more or less. People [didn't] actually speak about religious ethics per se. Then, as years go by, I noticed that more and more people are getting more interested ... jumping into the bandwagon of bioethical discourse and medical ethics discourse. There is a growing number of people who are looking at ethical issues from the religious perspective ... Today we see that the number of researchers ... looking into these issues [is growing] as well. Even if you look at the literature in international publications around the world, there has been a growing number of academic journals on religious ethics.

I'm not really sure how things developed to what they are today, but, of course, to me there is much room for improvement. There are many things to do, actually. One of the things, one of the problems today, is that whenever there is a scientific development or there is a new medical technology, for instance, we see that ethics is trying to catch up. When I say ethics, I'm referring to the secular ethics. The Islamic or religious ethics [is] even further behind. More often than that, we find technologies being developed at a very rapid rate. We are unable to cope with the rapid development in terms of looking at these developments from the ethical perspective, what more [the] religious perspective. I think that's one great challenge that we have to face.

(Malaysia Interview 32, "bridge" scholar, REC member)

The participant argues that it is very difficult for scientists/researchers to be fully aware of ethico-legal problems that may arise and for traditional scholars to be sufficiently versed in the complexities of emerging biomedical sciences. He therefore argues for the need for "bridge scholarship" – where a person can understand enough of the science but also be sufficiently aware of Islamic ethical issues. From the above quote, it is clear that the bridge-scholar has concerns about traditional scholars being able to provide contemporaneous advice from a religious perspective on rapidly emerging biomedical issues. He also explained the motivation for pursuing "bridge scholarship" and how efforts are being made in Malaysia to train more professionals to acquire dual specialism:

There are a number of challenges. Number one is that development in science and medicine is being done by people in science and medicine. Then those who talk about ethics, who talk about religious ethics, ... most of them, not all, but most of them do not have that background. They in essence speak two different languages ... What we need is actually a bridge to link these two groups. When I say bridge, here, I don't like to use the word hybrid, but more or less what I'm trying to say is we need somebody who is familiar with both areas, both the sciences and also the religious studies. Here at the Academy of Islamic Studies, we are actually developing that. For the past 13 years we have [had] a program called Islamic Studies and Science ... the students actually do a double major program. One major is on Islamic Studies. The other major is done at the faculty of Science.

These students, when they graduate, one of their advantages, and I've seen that with the graduates who have been produced before, one of the advantages is that they go into any lines they like. Some actually end[ed] up in the scientific community, some ended up in religious bodies and some ended up doing work to get the two together. I think that's the start, but the number is very small at the moment. If we can create these people who can speak the two languages, I think that can help a lot.

(Malaysia Interview 32, "bridge" scholar, REC member)

His experience and the experiences of other participants highlight a tension in the role of Islamic scholars in bioethics. Although their involvement, in both countries, has broadly been flexible and permissive of biomedical advancement, as seen in the example of stem cells above, the technical nature of biomedicine and its religio-ethical implications has not only forced discussions around issues relating to Islamic law and theology, but it is also challenging the traditional role and authority of Islamic scholars. The data analysis here also reveals that in Malaysia there is consideration for formally training scientists to be able to adequately engage in the process of Islamic ethico-legal reasoning. It suggests a distinctive role for so-called "bridge scholars" that is becoming more formally recognised than that seen for so-called contextual scholars. The latter are biomedical experts who may have personally undertaken training in the Islamic sciences, but they are not formally recognised as Islamic scholars.

Contextual scholars (biomedical experts) and evolving tensions in Islamic scholarly authority within biomedical research ethics in Malaysia and Iran

From the above discussions, it seems that in both countries Islamic scholars are looked upon to provide religious rulings either through legal or political require-ments or from personal need. However, beyond legal, national and/or Islamic legitimacy, do scholars add to the ethico-legal debate in Malaysia and Iran? Or, is their involvement simply for cultural appropriateness or for retaining traditional authority? In Malaysia, for example, one researcher, acting as a contextual scholar (one who provides information about the biomedical context), explained how he was asked to provide a specialist opinion to the National *Fatwah* Council on the public health benefits of researching and implementing a needle exchange pro-gramme and to assess the need for researching and administering porcine-based vaccines. Intravenous drug use and the consumption of porcine products are ille-gal in Islam, and the approval of researching such interventions was considered sensitive both for the research and clinical context. He shared the challenges he faced in convincing the Council about the benefits of such interventions, and the counter arguments he encountered in their commitment to retaining their authority and remaining "conservative" on such issues:

RESEARCHER/REC MEMBER: [T]he methadone, exchange of syringes, at one time it was very difficult to convince the *Fatwah* Council of the safety. They say, "[The] exchange of needles is encouraging the drug habit." ... Some of my colleagues say that it's a waste of time speaking to *Fatwah* Council, because they'll say, "Anything that's got pork no, no." You know vaccines, I'm a proponent of vaccines. I go around the country on a roadshow talking about vaccines, and now that's a big issue because of porcine in vaccines. So I said, "This is an issue that has been sorted out since the early 80s or 90s." ... I actually told them, "This is from the heart; I'm telling you, your *Fatawah* are conservative. Your *Fatwah* [are] out of date."

INTERVIEWER: Why is that? Why is there such a commitment to remain conservative?

RESEARCHER/REC MEMBER: I don't know. I think this is still a problem we have to deal with in Malaysia, and if you don't have the title of "scholar" before your name, it's very difficult for you to say. But I actually have to go beyond this, I have to champion it, *la*. I have spoken before the committees on various of these issues. I don't know why; it's just we have to wait for the new generation of scholars to come along and hopefully things will change.

(Malaysia Interview 30, Researcher, REC member)

The above indicates that, although traditional scholars are becoming more dependent on the technical evidence provided by biomedical experts who themselves are considerably well versed in the Islamic ethico-legal tradition, the "scholar" label is reserved for those trained in the traditional Islamic legal system. The religio-ethical deliberations may be carried out by traditional scholars and biomedical experts, however, the former are the ones who retain the authority of making the final decision on "what ought to be done" and "what ought to be approved" as being "Islamic".

The data analysis of the interviews conducted suggests that when issues that are considered relevant to Islamic law and theology emerge, in both countries Islamic scholars are consulted to review whether there is instruction within the normative sources of Islam (*Qur'an, Hadith, Shariah*, legal precedent in courts, *fatawah*) to direct what ought to be done. If there is no answer in the latter sources, then the scholars are required to undertake independent reasoning, or *ijtihad*, which is a process that incorporates two components to enable them to arrive at a *fatwah*. The first component for *ijtihad* is the contextual information about what the ethico-legal issue is, how it has arisen and what its implications may be, e.g., contextual information regarding stem cell research. The second component is the review of the overall values and instructions that Islamic scholars glean from Islam's normative sources to ensure that they arrive at an ethico-legal instruction (*fatwah*) about what ought to be done in light of Islam's normative sources, e.g., whether or not stem cell research can be approved.

Previously, biomedical researchers were expected to only provide the contextual information to enable Islamic scholars to then carry out *ijithad* to arrive at a legal edict (*fatwah*) on what ought to be done in relation to a given question/issue. Hence they are referred to as contextual scholars in the literature (Ramadan, 2008, p. 4). However, as the data analysis and previous two quotes reveal, and as will become evident in subsequent sections and chapters, biomedical experts (either as contextual or bridge scholars) within the context of research are becoming involved in both parts of this practical reasoning process. They provide the contextual information, and they have also been equipping themselves with the language and knowledge of the Islamic sciences to contribute to the second component, or the consideration of what the Islamic normative sources would instruct.

Additionally, in Iran one of the participants explained that the use of Islamic normative sources and the involvement of scholars are driven by researchers to provide validity to their work, rather than initiating/ensuring a rigorous academic discussion about the religio-ethico-legal soundness of interventions:

I think many researcher[s], many writer[s], they use *Qur'an* and *Hadiths* as they want. Even when they're asking Islamic scholars, they don't present whole the problem. There's no open discussion among scientist[s] and Islamic scholars. When [we're] trying to ask them [for] their comments, ... we just write them, send it, and they answer it in one sentence, and that's not helpful. ... [W]e have to make a scientific discussion between scientist[s] and Islamic scholars, to make clear the problem for them, and they could answer. They could research. And then, to find the real answer of the Islam, that's a big problem for us too. Some writers, some authors try to find the answer through the *Qur'an* and *Hadith* by themselves. Some of them ask the questions from a scholar as they want, as they need to find the answer, and that's the problem, that's not the Islam.

(Iran Interview 13, Researcher, REC member, guideline developer)

Her experience reveals a critical question in relation to this evolving scholarly authority in Islam. If traditional scholars are becoming more reliant on contextual scholars to provide the necessary information to enable them to make an ethico-legal decision through the process of *ijtihad*, what happens when the contextual scholars provide incomplete material? If such omission or manipulation is intentional, then what are the religio-ethico-legal implications of such a decision-making process and the end decisions (*fatawah*)? Chapter 8 will provide an exploration of the implications of such tensions on the broader Islamic bioethics discourse in terms of the process of *ijtihad* as a means of practical deliberation in arriving at an instruction on what ought to be done through the issuing of *fatawah*.

The above highlights that there are similarities and differences in the approaches to complexities arising from scholarly authority in both countries. Although there is religious oversight in Iran and researchers are required to grapple with this legal requirement, such as the mandatory membership of Islamic scholars within RECs, the absence of such a prescribed system results in equally challenging complexities in Malaysia, where personal religious reservations are witnessed within RECs and/ or researchers find themselves faced with "conservative" views within the National *Fatwah* Council.

However, as described in this chapter, these structures also display considerable flexibility as those involved encounter and address issues on a case-by-case basis. Overall, the experience of participants, analysed in this study, highlights that the elements of Islam that are relevant within discussions around biomedical research ethics are broadly flexible and permissive, however, there are complexities and constraints around religious authority and involving particular issues that have legal and/or theological implications within Islam, which will be discussed in Chapter 4.

Traditionally, Islamic scholars have been offered complete authority to arrive at an understanding and instruction of what ought to be done, where the consideration of Islamic values and law is deemed pertinent. This chapter, however, suggests that due to the technical nature of biomedical research and its implications for Islamic theology and law, scholars and researchers alike have been forced into deliberations about what ought to be done in particular contexts. This mechanism of practical reasoning involving *ijtihad* to produce *fatawah* is seeing an increasing role for biomedical experts and is creating a tension in what has been recognised traditionally as Islamic scholarly authority. Although this has been previously documented within the broader Islamic bioethics discussion (Ghaly, 2013), this research provides an example of such experiences and tensions within biomedical research.

Centres for Islamic bioethics in Iran and Malaysia

Seminaries in Qum and the MEHRC as emerging centres of Islamic bioethics in Iran

A traditional scholar based at the seminary in Qum explained how biomedical ethics is an emerging field of research in Iran and how he became involved in addressing emerging issues arising in the field:

> We focus on the bioethics because, here in Iran ... during [the] last more than ten years ..., we had some movement about bioethics, and there [were] many questions and many asking about our studies and our ideas in Islam about bioethics. So, we refer to this discipline because it has many request[s], and after we focused on this discipline, we saw that the area is very vast. And it covers mostly all of the area of applied ethics, because the field of living good and the health care – about the environment also, in some meaning – it's under this area ... You know that in Iran medicine is very fast in developing. They have many questions about the profession of medicine, about the relation between physician and patients and also questions about the medical researches, new researches ... Because our society is an Islamic society, the culture has very special influence on ethical studies. Our physicians, our people in Iran, our studies in Iran are asking about what Islam says about this kind of research. So it's important to consider this for the inner (Iranian) culture. For the outer culture also. When you go to any place for research, for addressing ... these areas, they are looking at you as an Islamic thinker. For example, in US they know the answer of Beauchamp and Childress. They want from me or you that you answer [a] different answer that comes from religion, that comes from your religion. What is *Shia* Islam's answer for this question?
>
> (Iran Interview 16, traditional scholar involved in national bioethics)

The scholar highlights that, for Iranian society, it is important for emerging biotechnology and research to be assessed by scholars in order for them to produce a *Shi'i* perspective on their acceptability and ethico-legal boundaries. He also emphasised how the international community looks to scholars like him to provide a *Shi'i* perspective on bioethical issues. He mentioned how the department of medical ethics at the seminary is in its nascent phase, but there is support from the government and demand from professionals, research ethics committees and the wider public to develop a *Shi'i* response to emerging bioethical issues, particularly around biomedical research.

Another traditional scholar explained how he has been employed by the Tehran University of Medical Sciences (TUMS) and the MOHME for several years to engage with bioethical questions to enable the development of decisions and guidelines that are religio-ethically acceptable:

> I'm cooperating with Ministry of Health at the same field, which is related to medical ethics ... actually in [the] medical science system ... departments and groups ... I mean the groups that are doing researches on medical ethics issues ... I'm one of the member[s] of this group ... Usually, [the] kind of questions ... in this group are about, "Is this research according to Islamic *Fiqh* (jurisprudence)?", and the source of ethics in my religion, mostly is in this field ... whether the researches could be evaluated based on Islamic ethics values. It means I'm looking for this in medical ethics committee. For example, research about humans, if this research is according to [the] value [s] of Islam ... for instance ... based on correct informing or harm avoidance principle[s] based on Islam religion. Has [this] been observed in this research or not?
>
> (Iran Interview 17, traditional scholar involved in national bioethics and REC)

The scholar explained how it was his remit to define benefits and harms of research proposals from an Islamic perspective to ensure that the research proposals are religio-ethico-legally acceptable. The ethico-legal deliberation of principles, such as benefits and harms from the Islamic perspective, will be further explored in Chapter 4.

MEHRC,[3] an academic department within TUMS is, also another site for specialisation in Islamic bioethics in Iran. The department is a collaboration of medical experts, Islamic legal scholars, bioethicists and researchers. It is an academic department that is responsible for producing national guidelines as well as publications that engage with the broader global bioethics discourse.

The Institute of Islamic Understanding (IKIM) – a government funded department developing Islamic ethics in Malaysia

Although Islam's institutional aspects are not systemically embedded within the bioethics infrastructure in Malaysia, as is seen in Iran, some of the participants explained the emerging role of a government-sponsored department in the development of the Islamic bioethics discourse in Malaysia. One of the participants explained how the Islamic bioethical discourse in Malaysia began through this department:

---

3 Tehran University of Medical Sciences. (2015). Department of Medical Ethics. http://gsia.tums.ac.ir/en/page/16696/Department-of-Medical-Ethics (Last accessed 30 March 2020).

I'm not really sure how that started, actually, but the discussion was initiated mainly by the Institute of Islamic Understanding Malaysia (IKIM) in the late 90s. The institute has actually published a number of books on ethics looking at scientific issues from Islamic ethics. I think that's when, probably, people started to take note of these issues.

(Malaysia Interview 32, "bridge" scholar, REC member)

The participant highlights a very important recent trend in Malaysia. There is an increasing interest within academic circles to incorporate Islamic ethical thinking. Although the formal structures, such as the Qum seminaries, are absent in Malaysia, Islamic ethics does find a place more recently in a government-funded department. IKIM's role in Islamic ethics/bioethics, however, is not very well described, and the publications to date are focused primarily on legal edicts (*fatawah*) rather than engaging with the broader global discussions on bioethics carried out by centres in Iran.

Role of Shariah, fiqh, ijtihad *and* fatawah *within the bioethical discourse in Malaysia and Iran*

As Islamic law (*Shariah*) is imbedded within the Iranian legal system, the function of the *Shariah* is integral to the judiciary and not within a parallel system as observed in Malaysia. One participant described how scholars, using the principles of Islamic jurisprudence (*fiqh*), address emerging issues and, because the *Shariah* is the prevailing legal system in Iran, the decisions that emerge become integral to national guidance and policy:

[W]e have something in our religion about some of those problems that have been appeared recently ... Our clergy are ready to start a deep study and make some solution from this.

(Iran Interview 2, national bioethics guideline developer)

The constitutional religion in Malaysia is Islam, with some authors suggesting that for Muslims it is the "ultimate source of ethics, morality, civilisation and everything else of value" (Nur, 2006, p. 223). Muslims in Malaysia are keen, therefore, to follow the guidance offered by Islam through the *Shariah* and the rulings of Islamic scholars, through the process of *ijtihad* in arriving at *fatawah*, the collections of which are compiled within works of Islamic jurisprudence or *fiqh*. This is indicated through the growing body of *fatawah* being issued in Malaysia on bioethical issues, such as including organ transplantation.[4] However, unlike Iran, Islamic law finds its place within a parallel system of state-level *Shariah* courts or the federal National *Fatwah* Council in Malaysia. This parallel system enables

---

4   Ministry of Health Malaysia. (2011). Organ transplantation from the Islamic perspective. http://www.moh.gov.my/moh/resources/auto%20download%20images/589d7ab14fcd6.pdf (Last accessed 24 March 2020).

flexibility where Islam and its sources can be called upon when needed, however, it also introduces challenges in terms of the lack of production of clear guidance and an in-built variation in state-level rulings, which can lead to injustices and inconsistencies in legal rulings and sentences. Such inconsistency is rarely found in Iran due to the nationalised *Shariah* system and a clearly demarcated hierarchy of Islamic authority.

Participants in Malaysia were asked about the role of Islamic scholarly *ijtihad*, the subsequent issuing of *fatawah*, the implementation of the *Shariah* and the remit of the *Shariah* courts within their own work. Their views highlight that the role of these elements is complex, as it results in a system where one set of rules are applied to Muslims and another applied to the rest of the population. For example, research on embryos has been debated recently in Malaysia, with Muslim scholars endorsing the use of embryos, as the common view amongst Muslim jurists is that ensoulment occurs at 120 days (Ghaly, 2012). One participant explained how the process of *ijtihad* about this issue and the new *fatwah* permits the use of embryos from Muslim couples for research:

> For example, one of them is in terms of the use of, in formulating the guide-lines for stem cell research, the source of cells. There's an issue about the use of the leftover embryos from in vitro fertilization, because Malaysia is multi-ethnic ... most in the population are the Malays. We also have the Indians, the Chinese. Of course, you have the varied regulation by other countries. We needed to do that because there was already application by some researchers to use leftover embryos. We actually had a meeting with the Muslim jurists, the National Fatwa Council, to discuss this, the use of leftover embryos by Muslim couples only. The non-Muslim couples, there are difficult issues there. Christians believe at fertilization life begins, whereas Muslims believe ensoulment begins at 120 days.
>
> When we faced the Muslim jurists, yes, finally the conclusion was it is per-missible to use leftover embryos for research, provided that the couple has agreed that they do not need any more of those embryos. They've completed their family. They already have twins, triplets, or a child. They want to donate that for research. That was one that had a religious bearing on it. This is so simple because in Islam, as you know, the benefit over harm, the benefit for mankind. Simple to achieve.
>
> (Malaysia Interview 18, Researcher, REC member)

When asked what action would take place if the guidance was breached, the researcher explained that as it relates to an Islamic ruling it would be covered by the *Shariah* court:

> I think the *Shariah* court, I'm sure there is a provision for that provided, again, there is a report. They can take action. If it's a Muslim doctor, yes, performing this, you can go to the *Shariah* track. Sometimes when you come

into something Muslim, that means the civil court can take action, but there are some cases when the *Shariah* court can come in as well.

(Malaysia Interview 18, Researcher, REC member)

However, he explained that such action required reporting about breaches, and these happened infrequently. Another layer of complexity emerges if a non-Muslim researcher misuses embryos that are donated by Muslim couples. Such malpractice would be covered by the federal system. However, the latter has a different penal system to the *Shariah* courts with the ability to confer harsher punishments.

Motivations for seeking fatawah

The data analysis of the interviews conducted suggests that when ethico-legal issues arise, researchers, REC members and guideline developers who are keen to make decisions that are harmonious with the Islamic faith, may consult traditional Islamic authority in the form of Islamic scholars, who either act as judges in the *Shariah* courts, within bodies that produce legal edicts (*fatwah* councils), or as individual scholars who issue *fatawah* (legal edicts) after undertaking *ijtihad* (independent reasoning). Islamic scholars either consider whether there is direct instruction from Islam's normative texts about what ought to be done, or they have to independently reason what is ethico-legally appropriate in light of these sources. Unsurprisingly, as has been shown from a literature review (Suleman, 2016), the *Qur'an, Hadith, Shariah* and existing books of jurisprudence (*fiqh*), do not provide a linear guide to bioethical decision-making. Rather, what scholars are tasked with is deliberation around ethico-legal issues as and when they emerge from biomedical research, through the process of *ijtihad* to produce instruction in the form of *fatawah*.

In both countries, the seeking of *fatawah* or religious edicts was for personal guidance as well as to ensure acceptance of an innovative method/therapy within the research context. One of the Islamic scholars in Malaysia explained that RECs refer to him or to other scholars for *fatawah*, as they worry they do not have the necessary religious credentials to make such decisions, nor are they willing to approve something that may be considered illegal from the perspective of the *Shariah*:

> The problem is the committee thinks that if they approve something which is prohibited, they are responsible for that [chuckles]. If they approve something, which is prohibited by Islam, the sin goes to them. That is why, the problem.

(Malaysia Interview 27, Muslim scholar REC member)

This notion of sin or moral accountability will be explored in more detail in Chapter 7.

In Iran, a researcher and REC member explained that being able to refer to a scholar or having them within the ethics committee is of great advantage as it enables the researchers and REC members to have the reassurance that they are conducting/approving studies and methods that are religio-legally acceptable:

> He may usually answer some questions, help us, mention some point to us. It's good. It's important ... for example, the *fatawah*, about stem cells, about embryonic studies, they help us to develop research in some fields ... As I remember, when stem cell study began, in all of the academic community, scientific community, it was an important question. It was a hot question. Can we go through this question or not? And I think Islamic Rouhanis (scholars) are very open-minded in scientific inquiry and know more about how the creation works. I think it's our chance that we have *fatwah*, and we can do our research with *itminan* (satisfaction) and *aramesh* (wellness).
>
> (Iran Interview 10, Researcher, REC member)

Another researcher, however, explained that the role of *fatawah* is to simply provide reassurance to society that the work being done by researchers is "Islamically" acceptable:

> *Fatwah* was not important for me. It's important for society, you know? I can understand what *Holy Qur'an* says, but they don't believe me. They believe clergymen, so I get *fatwah* to prove to the society that it's not a bad word, or it's not against Islam.
>
> (Iran Interview 5, Researcher, REC member, guideline developer)

Conclusions

In summary, this chapter has presented, from the interviews conducted, an analysis of the array of Islam's institutional aspects in Malaysia and Iran that are involved in the understanding of ethical issues in biomedical research. Firstly, this chapter highlights that issues relating to Islam are raised at multiple levels. They are addressed more centrally in Iran, due to the political establishment of an Islamic state, and through a parallel system in Malaysia, via state-level *Shariah* courts, national/state-level *fatwah* councils and/or individually consulted Islamic scholars (*muftis*). Secondly, this chapter also proposes that the elements of Islam and its normative sources that influence ethical thinking within biomedical research are not limited to, but include the foundational texts (*Qur'an* and *Hadith*), the *Shariah* (Islamic law), *fiqh* (Islamic jurisprudence), *ijtihad* (independent reasoning) to arrive at *fatawah* (legal edicts) and the involvement of Islamic scholars. When an ethico-legal issue emerges, the latter are tasked with interpreting Islam's foundational texts and law to provide instruction on what ought to be done through the unique process of *ijithad* in the development of *fatawah*. Thirdly, this chapter emphasises that the adaptability of Islam's institutional elements in the consideration of ethical issues in research in the case study sites shows that the overall system, though not predicable, works to meet the demands of those within it in a pragmatic and innovative fashion. Finally, the chapter also highlights that, although the involvement of Islamic scholars and the instruction derived from Islam's normative sources has been largely flexible and permissive, there are constraints and complexities that emerge around the issue of Islamic scholarly authority.

As explained above, although the task of *ijtihad* and issuing *fatawah* has been seen traditionally as the role of Islamic scholars, one of the striking features of the data analysis is that there is increasing involvement from biomedical experts (contextual scholars who are also informally trained in the Islamic sciences) and "bridge-scholars" (those formally being trained in biomedicine and the Islamic sciences), in the context of research and in this practical reasoning process. The latter and former provide contextual information, and they also have been equipping themselves with the language and knowledge of the Islamic sciences to contribute to the second component, or the consideration of what the Islamic normative sources would instruct. The data analysis also highlights that the label and recognition of Islamic scholarly authority is still reserved for those trained formally in the Islamic sciences. Although briefly explored here, a further discussion of the tensions and challenges arising from this evolution of Islamic scholarly authority, and how these three types of scholars have to work together in practice to resolve the dilemmas they encounter within the context of biomedical research, will be considered in Chapters 6 and 7.

Bibliography

Aghajanian, A. & Merhyar, A. H. (1999). Fertility, contraceptive use and family planning program activity in the Islamic Republic of Iran. *International Family Planning Perspectives*, 25(2), 98–102.

Ghaly, M. (2012). The beginning of human life: Islamic bioethical perspectives. *Zygon®*, 47(1), 175–213.

Ghaly, M. (2013a). Collective religio-scientific discussions on Islam and HIV/AIDS: I. Biomedical scientists. *Zygon®*, 48(3), 671–708.

Larijani, B., Zahedi, F. & Malek-Afzali, H. (2005). Medical ethics in the Islamic Republic of Iran. *East Mediterr Health J*, 11(5–6), 1061–1072.

Nur, S. N. M. (2006). The ethics of human cloning: With reference to the Malaysian bioethical discourse (pp. 215–246). In H. Roetz (Ed.). *Cross-cultural issues in bioethics: The example of human cloning* (Vol. 27). Amsterdam, The Netherlands: Rodopi.

Ramadan, T. (2009). *Radical reform: Islamic ethics and liberation*. New York: Oxford University Press.

Suleman, M. (2016). Contributions and ambiguities in Islamic research ethics and research conducted in Muslim contexts: I – A thematic review of the literature. *Journal of Health and Culture*, 1(1), 46–57.

Yusuf, A. (2014). Ethical issues in research ethics governance and their application to the Malaysian context. DPhil thesis. University of Oxford.

4 Islamic responses to the ethical issues of HIV/AIDS

Deeper analysis of the role of *ijtihad* and *fatawah* in the context of global health research ethics

The previous chapter provided an analysis of how the institutional forms of Islam in Malaysia and Iran influence ethical deliberations within biomedical research. Another important theme arising in my analysis of the interviews is that these institutional forms of Islam and the individuals within them face pressures of global health and global health policy. An analysis of how the institutional forms of Islam distinctly deal with such challenges is presented in this chapter. There have been calls for the "need to communicate what is shared and what is distinctive about Islamic perspectives and positions" (Childress, 2009, p. viii) in bioethics, and this chapter is an attempt at addressing this need.

For example, a key area of global health policy that is encountered in Malaysia and Iran is the HIV/AIDS epidemic. My data analysis shows that the ethical issues arising from HIV/AIDS require Islamic responses, as the epidemic raises issues about behavioural practices that are illegal in Islam. The institutional forms of Islam are formally employed to address the ethical issues of HIV/AIDS, and, in particular, Islamic scholars are trying to address the ethical issues through the process of *ijtihad* to derive *fatawah*. This mechanism of ethico-legal analysis has been employed in both Malaysia and Iran to support the research and health needs of intravenous drug users (IVDUs) through the approval of needle exchange programmes. However, the data analysis also shows that this mechanism is not as comprehensively employed in dealing with the challenges arising from the health needs of sex workers and men who have sex with men (MSM).

The global health challenge of curbing the spread of HIV/AIDS poses questions for the institutional forms of Islam

The global health challenge of curbing the spread of HIV/AIDS in Malaysia and Iran has raised questions about how the disease is spread and how the epidemic ought to be studied and managed. As HIV/AIDS is prevalent among marginalised groups, such as IVDUs, sex workers and MSMs, understanding the epidemiological trends in such groups and meeting their health needs has been challenging.

Religious and ethical concerns about the investigation of illicit practices

The data analysis indicates that there are religious concerns about investigating and addressing methods of HIV spread. IV drug use, sex work and homosexuality are all illegal in Islam. Participants explained that researching such communities without making an attempt at preventing such behaviours and supporting the distribution of condoms and needle exchange programmes would only perpetuate such illegal activities. One participant in Malaysia explained the challenge of researching marginalised groups:

> If those research questions are asking very obviously *haram* [illegal in Islam] questions, no ethics committee will entertain it, because it's socially and religiously insensitive ... such research may have been done by researchers in [the] School of Social Science, psycholog[y] and whatnot, and I believe they probably have done it. If you go to some groups of social scientists, they are very active in research into LGBT issues, transgender and whatnot. They probably are the best persons to ask, but I don't think that their protocol is being approved by any ethics committee. They probably just do it as part of social research, but it's a moot point. I keep telling people that anytime ... the religion is involved, anytime there's direct human contact involved, you must at least return the protocol to ethics committee. It may be given an ethical waver, but it must be seen by independent person – and I think some people actually don't do that, especially when it comes to social research.
>
> (Malaysia Interview 21, Researcher, REC member)

The participant explained and the data analysis indicates that there have been growing concerns that social science researchers are conducting research on such areas without ethics approval. The latter may be able to carry out the research, but they face problems when publishing and disseminating the results due to the absence of ethics approval and the potential political backlash from circulating data that is deemed unfavourable.

A variation in views about how to research and address the HIV/AIDS epidemic

My analysis of the data shows that issues that are illegal from the perspective of the *Shariah* require greater scrutiny and consideration by the RECs in Iran and Malaysia due to their illicit nature and the potential impact of the dissemination of research findings to the wider public and political authority. Participants explained that research on, for example, extramarital relationships is problematic, as researching such topics implies the acceptance of such activities. The data analysis reveals that in both countries there were similar differences in views when participants were asked about the scale of the HIV/AIDS burden and the acceptance and uptake of research and prevention programmes for HIV/AIDS amongst sex workers, MSMs and IVDUs. These views include those who considered the problem as being absent in a Muslim majority country; those who accepted that the burden of disease existed and ought to be tackled, but primarily using methods that emphasised abstinence and a removal of "unIslamic practices"; and those who considered it a professional responsibility to tackle the HIV/AIDS epidemic and considered the religious concerns as secondary.

Denial about HIV/AIDS being prevalent in Muslim countries is illustrated by:

> We have not HIV problem. HIV problem, it is due to that type of western-type freedom that produces HIV problem. Now, we should think about how to solve this problem. Most of the Islamic principle has the role of the prevention. Most of the ethical problem in the US and western countr[ies] is a type of treatment. Prevention is more important than treatment. We should start doing some of those good principles that prevent the society from this type of bad ethical point.
>
> (Iran Interview 2, Researcher, REC member, guideline developer)

Prevention being key to curtailing the HIV/AIDS epidemic is illustrated by:

> I've been involved with the Islamic Medical Association. We have discussed this. Again, most of the Muslims believe, yes, you must address the root of the problem. You cannot just ... Because of your objective, then you make the means *halal*. If your objective is to reduce the prevalence of HIV or STD or whatever, but you condone the use of protection, the use of condoms, the use of exchange of needles, that means that drug use itself is *haram*. But now you say you're going to allow. That means in Islam, all we've been taught to tackle the root of problems. That means by educating our teenagers on the bad effects on drug abuse and non-protected sex, and all this.
>
> (Malaysia Interview 18, Researcher, REC member)

Professional duty to researching the problem and providing healthcare being key is illustrated by:

> Because my responsibility is defined with the health services. My responsibility is not in the religious, so I have to help the people, even the prostitute, to be healthy and to keep safe. I have to provide the best health services, including OCPs, including condom, etc., because I am responsible.
>
> (Iran Interview 12, Researcher, REC member)

> I wear more of my doctor hat in this case, and [my] public health hat and my role is not to tell them to be a good Muslim, my role is to tell them how to protect themselves and that's it, simple.
>
> (Malaysia Interview 29, Researcher, REC member)

It is important to highlight that many healthcare professionals in Malaysia are affiliated to, lead and support the Federation of Islamic Medical Associations

(FIMA). Many of the respondents cited FIMA as a source of Islamic ethico-legal guidance (FIMA, 2015).[1] In August 2015, FIMA released the following statements:

> WHEREAS in the Islamic paradigm, HIV/AIDS is not considered as just a virus-induced disease, but rather a manifestation of a serious breakdown of socio-moral and behavioural norms afflicting human societies at varying degrees.
>
> (FIMA Admin, 2015)

> FIMA training and public awareness activities utilized latest scientific advances and epidemiologic knowledge, side-by-side with Islamic teachings and guidance that advocate values of self-discipline, chastity, morality, decency, family centricity, and reject the expanding trends of promiscuity, homosexuality, commercial sex, drug abuse and other behaviours, that will always undermine global efforts to effectively combat the HIV/AIDS pandemic.
>
> (FIMA Admin, 2015)

These tensions regarding the existence of illicit practices and what ought to be done to address the subsequent health needs have also been recorded in the literature in relation to other Muslim majority countries. For example, health problems linked to illicit practices, according to the *Shariah*, such as alcohol, drugs and extramarital sex, have resulted in disagreements about the distribution of publicly administered health resources and the funding and support for research in these areas (Sachedina & Ainuddin, 2004). It has been reported, as discussed in a literature review (Suleman, 2016), that health professionals, the public and scholars alike, in parts of the Muslim world, have considered those with HIV/AIDS as undeserving of healthcare resources (Ghaly, 2013a).

What is important to consider, however, is that, despite these differing views in Malaysia and Iran, concerted efforts are being made to tackle the HIV/AIDS epidemic with the involvement of Muslim scholars and the normative Islamic texts and legal tradition. It is also important to note that the process by which this ethico-legal negotiation occurs is not only distinctly Islamic, as it relies on Islamic textual sources and Islamic authority, but that the methods are distinct between the two countries due to their historically distinct theological-philosophical traditions. The mechanism that is employed by Islamic scholars to address the health needs arising from HIV/AIDS in the case of IVDUs will be considered in the

---

1 "The Federation of Islamic Medical Associations (FIMA) is a registered body of 29 IMAs (Islamic Medical Associations) and 17 associate members worldwide, representing about 50,000 Muslim medical and health professionals. The mission of FIMA is to provide a platform for Muslim Physicians world wide in the areas of Medical education and ethics, Student camps and humanitarian and medical relief. It is a not-for-profit, non-political and non-Governmental organization" (FIMA. (2015). Constitution. https://fimaweb.net/about-fima/constitution (Last accessed 22 August 2016)).

next section, and it offers a powerful example of the flexibility and permissiveness of the Islamic ethico-legal system.

The data analysis signifies that Islam's legal-theological boundary sets up tensions and questions for biomedical researchers, RECs, and guideline developers that require the involvement of scholars. Some of the issues that need to be deliberated include:

- What happens when there is disagreement or tension between what is instructed by Islamic law and global health pressures, as is seen when researching and addressing the spread of HIV/AIDS?
- Are illicit practices, such as IVDU and, therefore, needle exchange programmes, deemed categorically prohibited, such that any associated research and health policy strategies are restricted?
- Are the Islamic legal considerations for such issues suspended or reconsidered to enable a response to such emerging health needs?
- If there is flexibility, then is such concession applied across all illicit practices that impact health needs?
- Also, if the normative texts are considered clear in their guidance on the illicit nature of such issues, according to participants in this study, then what tools are used to engage in an ethico-legal analysis of such issues?

The data analysis presented in subsequent sections in relation to the ethical issues of HIV/AIDS research suggests that the empirical reality is complex and evolving in both countries.

The participants' views analysed in this study suggest that Islam's normative texts (*Qur'an* and *Hadith*) are clear in defining the illicit nature of the use of harmful substances, such as IV drugs, alcohol, extramarital sex and homosexuality. However, research on all of these issues and meeting the health needs of such groups is of professional and ethical importance to biomedical researchers. Does Islam offer a mechanism of dealing with such a tension? The process of *ijtihad* to derive *fatawah* is employed by Islamic scholars in Malaysia and Iran to address this tension.

Practical deliberation using *ijtihad* to derive *fatawah* as a mechanism of addressing ethical issues of HIV/AIDS

The previous chapter and the sections above reveal that, despite apparent socio-economic, geopolitical and theological differences in Malaysia and Iran, in both settings there is an empirically evident commitment to refer to Islamic authority when thinking about ethico-legal concerns emerging from biomedical research. What is "good research" in Muslim contexts? It is not simply about conducting effective and efficient research with ethical conduct – it also involves a deep spiritual and physical obligation to the teachings of Islam (this personal commitment to the Islamic faith will be explored in more detail in Chapter 6). Islam, therefore, adds an additional layer to the traditional understanding of "good research"

(Kerasidou & Parker, 2014) in these settings and relates to the "remarkable impact of the central grand narrative of Islam on the day-today lives of Muslims" (HRH The Prince of Wales, 2007, p. v). In both countries there has been, therefore, significant investment in establishing a structure (though different in both settings) for Islamic ethico-legal reference that is referred to when researchers, REC members and guideline developers encounter religio-cultural concerns. This section explores in more detail the complex relationship between the development of *fatawah*, the ethico-legal deliberations involved in the process of *ijtihad* and how these relate to the legal systems in Malaysia and Iran.

The relationship between Islamic texts, scholarship, interpretation and the lived experience of believers is a complex one. The discussion in Chapter 3 seems to suggest that there exists a complementarity between the issuing of *fatawah* with the consideration of ethical challenges and how they become binding in law. For example, the demand for researching an emerging reproductive technology may arise if the intervention overlaps or interferes with Islamic ethico-legal interests relating to the family, then such an intervention would be flagged by either scholars or researchers or practitioners and reviewed by the relevant religio-ethical authority. The latter would in turn issue a legal opinion or *fatwah* derived from a process of ethico-legal reasoning (*ijtihad*) that would not be legally binding but would confer, however, religious permissibility or impermissibility. As *fatawah* are legal opinions and not court rulings, they can be accepted or rejected, resulting in a plethora of *fatawah* for the same or similar ethico-legal questions. What appears an unsystematic and bewildering variation in views is an expression of ethico-legal plurality in Islam. Beyond the small range of unambiguous or prescribed duties found in the foundational texts of Islam, scholars are called upon to navigate the large spectrum of emerging concerns or revisit previously encountered problems that require a fresh approach.

The data in this study and subsequent analysis suggest that in both countries the process of *ijithad* to derive *fatawah* plays a significant role in stimulating or endorsing an ethical re-evaluation of emerging health issues that are perceived in a negative light due to their traditional legal status. It is an institutional mechanism of communication that is distinctive to Islam. This mechanism will be explored in more detail in relation to the ethical issues and health needs arising from the HIV/AIDS epidemic.

IVDUs and needle exchange programmes – a practical application of ijtihad and fatawah to address the ethical issues of HIV/AIDS

Employing the principle of public good (Maslaha) to address the ethical issues of HIV/AIDS in Iran

Ijtihad, as explained in Chapters 1 and 3, is a distinctly Islamic ethico-legal reasoning tool that involves two components. The first is understanding the contextual ethico-legal question, which is often provided by biomedical experts, and the second is engagement with Islam's normative sources to arrive at a consideration of the values and laws prescribed by the latter, which can result in a *fatwah* being issued. Participants explained that the letter of Islamic law in relation to IV drug use is clear – it is illegal. However, they mentioned that there are values that enable a broader understanding of Islam's law to allow a response to the health needs emerging from such illicit practices. One such value is that of ensuring "public good" that is deliberated through the Islamic ethico-legal principle of *Maslaha*.

Maslaha is the principle of "public interest" or "public good" that is taken into consideration when *fatawah* are derived through the process of *ijtihad*. *Maslaha* is an Islamic principle that takes into account the context with an emphasis that when the text is silent, you need to derive an understanding of the *Maslaha* or what is in the public's interest. Reflecting this Islamic ethico-legal process, a few participants in Iran explained how Iranian society and those in authority are becoming more aware and accepting of the health needs of marginalised groups, such as IVDUs, and they are thinking proactively about how to address these needs in a way that is coherent with their religio-cultural context. My data analysis indicates that, although IV drug use is illegal in Islam, the "public good" that would arise from researching and implementing a needle exchange programme for IVDUs, as a mechanism of curbing the spread of disease, is considered sufficiently important, and so applying the principle of *Maslaha* to lend approval to such an intervention is considered appropriate:

> The ethical issue remains about there still being problems and health needs in these marginalized groups, and how [do] we get around the problem of discussing ... I think when it comes to our society, the best way would be to conduct that research in a high-risk population ... We had this problem with our prisoners few years ago. It was really hard for many authorities in the country that we have to give them a syringe. They said if we distribute syringe to prisoners, that means they can have their addiction when they are in the prison, and they can have substances, drug abuse. But, finally, the health authority could convince them (Islamic scholars) that good comes out of this plan. It's better than ignoring the problem, and they accepted. They saw the result from research done here. The situation was better ... What I have seen with the prisoners, I can see the change. I can predict that for those type of issues, we will have the same change.
>
> (Iran Interview 15, national bioethics guideline developer)

The participant explained that there has been commitment from the health authority and biomedical professionals to inform Islamic scholars and the political authority about the health problems relating to HIV/AIDS, IVDU and the possible benefit from research and implementation of needle exchange programmes. This is despite the fact that such an intervention and the practice of IVDU is illegal in Islam. Subsequent to such discussions in Iran, in 2003 the government legalised needle exchange programmes, becoming one of the first countries in the region to do so (Mahdavi, 2008, pp. 1–50). The researcher did, however, explain that such a commitment did not change the boundary of Islamic law, as these practices are still considered outside the margins of the *Shariah*. Commentators have suggested that, since Khatami's presidency in the 1990s, the government has issued *fatawah* encouraging HIV research and has funded public-media campaigns (Mahdavi, 2008, pp. 1–50). Iran's experience of IVDUs and the implementation of needle exchange programmes highlight that, although the letter of the law is unchanged, the principle of "public good" can be applied to address the spread of HIV/AIDS.

Maqasid al-Shariah (The Higher Objectives of Islamic law) as a means of addressing the ethical issues of HIV/AIDS in Malaysia

The understanding and application of the Islamic principle of *Maslaha* is contested in Malaysia. Scholars in Malaysia question what is understood as "public good", are reluctant to simply accept an experiential understanding of "public good" and are committed to ensuring that such an understanding is still rooted in the normative texts (Shabana, 2014). The data reveal that many participants in Malaysia stressed that the boundaries of Islamic law, or what is considered lawful and unlawful, is a means of deciding "good" from "bad". In Iran, however, such definitions are taken more from experience than scripture. As explained in Chapter 1, this distinction is seen in the earlier centuries of Islam where the *Ash'ari* school of theology defined "good" and "bad" based upon the text, and they suggested that rationality be used when there is no text. As extramarital sex, IVDU and homosexuality are forbidden, interventions that overlook or potentially support such actions are not acceptable. The *Ash'ari* view is the one that is most commonly inherited by *Sunni* scholars in Malaysia. The *Mu'tazilis*, by contrast, define "good" and "bad" based upon rationality that is informed by scripture, and *Shi'i* scholars of Iran have more readily accepted their thinking. The *Ash'aris* claim that, if based on reason, definitions of "good" and "bad" may be subject to changeable cultural practices and beliefs. For example, extramarital relations were previously considered "bad" in parts of the world where such practices are now acceptable.

The *Ash'ari* emphasis on the ethico-legal boundary of Islam is reflected in the data analysis through the commitment expressed by the many Muslim researchers, REC members and guideline developers in Malaysia who were reluctant to engage in discussions relating to illicit practices and concerned about the possibility of condoning such practices. They emphasised that the means cannot be *haram* (illegal) even if the ends are considered "good". *Mu'tazilis* and those prioritising reason as a means of discerning right from wrong would not consider extramarital relations lawful, and they would not alter the *Shariah* stipulation regarding this issue. Rather, the consideration of the consequences relating to the spread of an epidemic and the availability of interventions to address such harms are given more weight in determining the appropriateness of whether HIV/AIDS research and prevention programmes can be implemented. It was not unusual for me to encounter Malaysian researchers or practitioners with decades of experience in biomedical practice and research who considered HIV/AIDS research and interventions, such as needle exchange programmes, problematic areas. A few of the participants in Malaysia considered the Islamic ethico-legal perspective as simply consisting of legal do's and don'ts and, therefore, relied on and expected scholars to provide such prescribed legal guidance.

The Malaysian experience reveals that healthcare professionals and pressure groups have faced resistance in putting together a response to the challenge of HIV/AIDS. One senior researcher in Malaysia explained that she had been working for a number of years on HIV/AIDS and, in particular, on research and prevention programmes for IVDUs and, more recently, for sex workers. Her research is considered taboo, and she has been questioned for condoning practices that are illicit according to Islamic law:

> I do a wide range of research focusing largely on HIV/AIDS, but also, just a little less, on general infectious disease ... and in HIV/AIDS, I couldn't choose. I mean HIV/AIDS is already controversial, but I couldn't choose to do more non-mainstreaming, in a sense that I do mostly research with the marginalized communities or in the HIV world. It's now called "key affected population". Initially, [we were] mostly focusing on drug users, prisoners. [N]ow, we're also branching into the sex workers and men who have sex with men, so all of the very tabooed, marginalized communities in this country and others ... We come across all the time, with needle exchange and all that, "You're condoning it".
>
> (Malaysia Interview 29, Researcher, REC member)

Another participant explained that, for Muslim jurists in Malaysia, it is important to ensure that both the means and ends of a public health intervention are in keeping with Islamic law:

> But the jurists, they'll look at it again. Because of the objectives, you cannot make the means *halal*. If the way itself is not right, you cannot make it permissible. You must tackle it at the bottom. I think that's the current climate of the jurists. That's why there's an opposition between the AIDS council, the patient group and the religious group, in terms of promotion of the exchange of needles, as well as telling teenagers sex education. For them, premarital sex is *haram*, an illegal couple. That is the approach. They're not meeting, anyway, because the belief is different.
>
> (Malaysia Interview 18, Researcher, REC member)

Given the pressures to reconcile what is stipulated by Islamic law and what participants considered ethically important from the biomedical profession in terms of researching and addressing HIV/AIDS rates, some of the participants in Malaysia explained that they considered it necessary to engage Islamic scholars regarding this issue. Islamic scholars who are engaging with these biomedical experts on HIV/AIDS in IVDUs have been found to be willing to consider the underlying objectives of the law, not simply the letter of the law, to address the latter group's health needs and to curb the spread of disease.

Many of the participants in Malaysia referred to a framework that is implemented within the process of *ijtihad* that is used to arrive at a locally acceptable understanding of *Maslaha*. As explained above, the understanding and application of the Islamic principle of *Maslaha* is contested in Malaysia. In Malaysia, the deployment of the higher objectives of the *Shariah* (*Maqasid al Shariah*) is used to develop the notion of *Maslaha* (see Chapter 1 for further information about the historical roots of the *Maqasid*). This is to ensure that an understanding of "public good" is not arbitrarily developed, rather it is still rooted in the normative texts (Shabana, 2014). The objectives that are used in Malaysia are that of "preservation of life" and "protection of progeny", where researching and implementing a needle exchange programme is deemed necessary as it protects life and prevents spread of disease to future generations. Although the *Maqasid* were developed to enable a response to ethico-legal issues independent of the normative texts, *Sunni* scholars, like those observed in Malaysia, have sought to prevent undisciplined employment of these objectives.

One of the participant's experiences highlights not only the influence of religious scholars in Malaysia, but also their keenness to implement the *Maqasid al-Shariah* within the process of *ijtihad*. What is also important to note is how healthcare professionals, who are keen to have Islamic ethico-legal frameworks that are simple and systematic to navigate through, readily understand and accept the *Maqasid*:

> Firstly, the majority of the drug users are Malays or Muslims; and secondly, quite a lot of the negative, the criticisms, came from religious scholars, other religious scholars. And, because they have a very influential voice, if they say "no", then the general public will also not approve and will create lots of problems for us. So, in fact, we did it as a pre-empt thing. Even before we went public, we had already consulted the religious scholars. They are [a] very powerful lot in this country.
>
> When we were setting up the needle exchange program, there was [a] huge debate. I was under ... attack in terms of precisely that, condoning drug use, which is considered *haram* (illegal according to Islamic law). The same with methadone – giving drug users methadone; just replacing one *haram* material with another. So, we did consult religious scholars, and that's where we used the dictum, "We're doing something [of] lesser evil for the greater good kind of thing[s].
>
> I worked very closely ... around the *Shariah* principles of protection of life, those five things of life. Progeny ... we argued [that] by preventing people from getting HIV, by giving them clean needles, ... you [are] saving their lives, you [are] saving their progeny, saving the world. What were the other two? Yeah, faith. Intellect, yeah ... It made complete and total sense to me; it was something very easy to understand and accept.
>
> (Malaysia Interview 29, Researcher, REC member)

Although the process by which *ijtihad* is undertaken and the underlying principles are distinct in Malaysia and Iran, scholars in both countries emphasised the need to uphold the underlying norms and values highlighted by the Islamic normative sources, such as public good and preservation of life.

In Malaysia and Iran, deliberations between professionals and scholars, through the process of *ijtihad* based on the principles of *Maqasid* or an understanding of *Maslaha* has uncovered a method of ethico-legal reasoning that may enable the reconciliation of biomedical concerns and global health pressures that involve interventions that are prohibited according to Islamic law. Although "the means", such as needle exchange, are *haram* (illegal) in these instances, such interventions can still be given religious endorsement based on the *Maqasid* or an understanding and application of *Maslaha*.

The discussion thus far may suggest that the flexible and permissive practical deliberation offered by *ijtihad* in deriving *fatawah* may be universally applied to address tensions raised by Islam's legal and theological boundaries. However, the next section shows that the reality is more complex, and this mechanism is not so easily formulated or applied for other issues that are illegal in Islam.

Researching and addressing HIV/AIDS in sex workers and the LGBT community

The data analysis shows that there is a difference seen in the two case study sites in terms of professionals being able to research and implement education and barrier contraception programmes for sex workers at risk of HIV/AIDS. One participant in Malaysia emphasised how the "religious conservatism" in Malaysia resulted in differences in policies and practices within the biomedical sciences compared with countries like Iran. He said the following in reference to carrying out research on marginalised groups, such as sex workers, in Malaysia:

> [I]n Malaysia, because of religious conservativ[ism], sex workers are not a recognised entity, but [they are] in some other Muslim countr[ies], including Bangladesh – I know this because a friend of mine is doing a study in Bangladesh ... They are organized. They['ve] got their own organisations, and, as such, research into sex workers – either social or cultural research, even commercial stud[ies] – is going on in these countries. I'm sure you'll find the same for Iran. Iran even has ... more of a liberal approach for this.
>
> (Malaysia Interview 21, Researcher, REC member)

Some participants in Iran explained how similar political sensitivities exist in Iran, where they planned to carry out research on sexually transmitted diseases (STDs), such as HIV/AIDS. However, a senior researcher in Iran explained that, unlike Malaysia, sensitive research can be more openly negotiated with religious authorities so long as the publication of data is carefully managed due to the religio-political sensitivities, including implications from international media:

I think that, here in this concern, you can say that the Iranian people and Iranian researchers are more open. In fact, there is the value of doing this research ... there [is] a lot of research in these fields, even [though] we know that it's illegal. It's not acceptable in terms of Islamic beliefs, and this country the Islamic state, with a lot of propaganda about this. But, we don't see the harshness about this in the field of research. It's possible to do this type of research if you regulate your relationship with authorities to get their licensed permission for doing the research. It's possible. It's not very difficult to do this research. You can see researchers on sex workers. It's illegal. It's not possible. But, I think that they accept it ... It exists, and even [though] sometimes they deny [it]. But, they accept that there is no solution, and [they] should accept some researchers in this field. We can see some researchers in the field of sex workers, etc., in this country.

Sometimes, because they want to keep bad things private, bad situations private, they don't like to share, because sometimes in international media, the small things get propaganda ... I think that we should publish this data with enough clarification. Without judgment. Usually, there is no problem to publish your data in Iran. Usually. I have evidence for it in the Middle East countries. Iran is among the few countries that publish their HIV numbers, AIDS numbers, very freely without any concern ... [In Iran] I think that people are religious, but they are open.

(Iran Interview 14, Researcher, REC member, guideline developer)

He explained that, although sensitive topics may require greater scrutiny, in terms of national politics, media and publication, as the lines of religious authority and expectations are clear, they can be negotiated because the religious authority is heavily invested in ensuring public good. In Malaysia such a clear line of religious authority does not exist, and some of the researchers' experiences captured here highlight that they feel they have to understand personally what Islam says and, therefore, try to uphold or protect views of the tradition.

In Malaysia the lesbian, gay, bisexual and transsexual (LGBT) communities face "stigma and discrimination" (Mahathir, 2013, p. 121), because they are considered to engage in behaviours that are "immoral" and "illegal" according to Islamic law (Mahathir, 2013, pp. 116–47). Although research is done in marginalised groups, many REC members expressed that they have and would continue to refuse to authorise such research, and many researchers expressed an unwillingness to conduct such studies. This is not simply due to these groups being hard to reach or publicly stigmatised, researchers and REC members themselves expressed an inability to reconcile their religious obligations in relation to these groups:

There are some discussions about, for example, doing research in homosexual, bisexual as well as transgender [groups]. I find ... It's been difficult for us to decide whether we should allow this kind of research, because I will say, "Why do you want to do [this kind of] research?" ... My concern is that if you do research ... we are allowing them to continue ... something that is against their religion, especially if you involved Muslim[s] ... If you are doing the research in the subject, who is actively involved and continuously involved? You are sort of allowing them to do something [that] is not acceptable. How are you going to answer for that?

(Malaysia Interview 26, Researcher, REC member)

Again, this notion of moral accountability expressed in the phrase "How are you going to answer for that?" will be explored in Chapter 6.

If you wanted to do a piece of research that looked at the prevalence of sexually transmitted diseases in the gay community, for example, or even working out their health needs, then is that something that you could do?
I think probably it would be difficult to get ethics [approval]. They may not stop [it], but to get the patients, to get the volunteers, I think that would be even harder. Nobody will dare to come out and say, "We are this group." Probably sex workers may not be that difficult, but this type of group (MSM), I think it will be more difficult for them to admit they are in that group.

(Malaysia Interview 34, Researcher, REC member)

A more detailed analysis of the tensions that arise for researchers trying to reconcile their personal and professional values in the case of HIV/AIDS research will be explored in more detail in Chapter 6. Here the focus is on how the institutional elements of Islam, particularly the process of *ijtihad* in deriving *fatawah*, are used to address the ethical challenges of HIV/AIDS. My data analysis suggests that, in addition to researchers' own tensions about how to reconcile the global health challenge and their own personal convictions, individuals from such marginalised groups would be reluctant to participate in such research due the risk of being identified as engaging in practices that are illegal in Islam and socio-culturally taboo.

Iran has deemed homosexual acts punishable by death (Kennedy, 2007) and has implemented what has been described as an "extreme" policy (Carter, 2010, p. 800) and *fatwah* of state-sponsored and subsidized "sex-change surgery as a means of the 'normalization' of homosexual men and women" (Carter, 2010, p. 797) who have been "diagnosed transsexuals" (Carter, 2010, p. 798). The policy points to ethico-legal concerns beyond HIV/AIDS to broader concerns around sexuality and sexual health in Iran. It is important to highlight that, given Iran is "a country with the highest death penalty enforcement per capita in the world and [the] second highest rate of sexual reassignment surgery" (Carter, 2010, p. 799), it underlines the extent to which health research and health resources are impacted by the State's concern to uphold its interpretation of Islamic law.

These challenges indicate that, although the process of *ijithad* and the issuing *fatawah* are a distinct and recognisably important means of ethico-legal deliberation in Islamic contexts, there may be variations in their application. This mechanism of ethico-legal analysis has been employed in both Malaysia and Iran to support the research and health needs of IVDUs through the approval of needle exchange programmes. However, the data analysis also shows that this mechanism is not as comprehensively employed in dealing with the challenges arising from the health needs of sex workers and MSMs. The data analysis suggests that it is not simply about some activities being illegal and, therefore, prohibited. Rather, issues like prostitution and homosexuality are more challenging than, for example, needle exchange programmes for IVDUs, as these practices are taboo and socio-culturally unacceptable.

Conclusions

In summary, this chapter has shown, firstly, that the institutional forms of Islam described in Chapter 3 and the individuals within them face pressures of global health and global health policy. For example, a key area of global health policy encountered in Malaysia and Iran is the HIV/AIDS epidemic. Secondly, my data analysis shows that the ethical issues arising from HIV/AIDS require Islamic responses, as the epidemic raises issues about behavioural practices that are illegal in Islam. Thirdly, my analysis indicates that the institutional forms of Islam are formally engaged with in order to address the ethical issues of HIV/AIDS. In particular, Islamic scholars are trying to address the ethical issues through the process of *ijtihad* to derive *fatawah*. This chapter offers a more substantive account of the ethical issues emerging from HIV/AIDS research, including how "public good" is understood through the process of *ijtihad* to derive *fatawah* in Malaysia and Iran to instruct researchers on what ought to be done in the case of IVDUs and needle exchange programmes. It suggests that the Islamic-ethico-legal system is flexible and permissive enough to deal with the tensions that arise as a result of pressures of global health and global health policy. It also presents this mechanism as being distinct in the two countries due to their theological-philosophical traditions. Finally, this chapter illustrates that, despite the permissive and flexible mechanism of practical deliberation offered by *ijtihad* in producing *fatawah*, there are tensions that still exist in the consideration of the health needs of sex workers and the LGBT community in Malaysia and Iran. My analysis of the data suggests that more work needs to be done to assess the role of the Islamic ethico-legal system in addressing such global health challenges and determine how certain issues may be dealt with differently due to their being taboo and socio-culturally unacceptable.

Bibliography

Carter, B. J. (2010). Removing the offending member: Iran and the sex-change or die option as the alternative to the death sentencing of homosexuals. *J. Gender Race & Just.*, 14, 797–832.

Childress, J. F. (2009). Forward. In A. Sachedina (Ed.). *Islamic biomedical ethics: Principles and application* (p. viii). New York: Oxford University Press.

FIMA. (2015). About FIMA. http://fimaweb.net/cms/index.php/about (Last accessed 22 August 2016).

FIMA Admin. (2015). FIMA declaration on global efforts to combat the HIV/AIDS pandemic. https://fimaweb.net/fima-declaration-on-global-efforts-to-combat-the-hiv-aids-pandemic (Last accessed 22 August 2016).

Ghaly, M. (2013a). Collective religio-scientific discussions on Islam and HIV/AIDS: I. Biomedical scientists. *Zygon®*, 48(3), 671–708.

HRH The Prince of Wales. (2007). Foreword. In A. Sheikh & A. R. Gatrad (Eds.). *Caring for Muslim patients*. New York: Radcliffe Publishing.

Kennedy, D. (2007). Gays should be hanged, says Iranian minister. *The Times*. http://www.timesonline.co.uk/tol/news/world/middle-east/article2859606.ece (Last accessed 22 August 2016).

Kerasidou, A. & Parker, M. (2014). Does science need bioethicists? Ethics and science collaboration in biomedical research. *Research Ethics*, 10(4), 214–226. doi:10.1177/1747016114554252.

Mahathir, M. (2013). *Telling it straight*. Singapore: Didier Millet Pte, Editions.

Mahdavi, P. (2008). *Passionate uprisings: Iran's sexual revolution*. Stanford, CA: Stanford University Press.

Sachedina, A. & Ainuddin, N. (2004). *Islamic biomedical ethics: Issues and resources*. Islamabad: COMSTECH.

Shabana, A. (2014). Bioethics in Islamic thought. *Religion Compass*, 8(11), 337–346.

Suleman, M. (2016). Contributions and ambiguities in Islamic research ethics and research conducted in Muslim contexts: I – A thematic review of the literature. *Journal of Health and Culture*, 1(1), 46–57.

5   Women and biomedical research ethics
Religion, culture and ethics

Chapter 3 looked at an analysis of the institutional forms of Islam that are involved in biomedical research ethics, and Chapter 4 examined how these institutional forms and the individuals within them face pressures of global health and global health policy, such as HIV/AIDS. Another important theme arising in my analysis of the interviews was that these institutional forms of Islam may be appropriated to support and/or maintain cultural views and practices.

It became evident from the literature review (Suleman, 2016) and also the analysis of early interviews in both Malaysia and Iran that the role and status of women in these contexts and their involvement in biomedical research was an important theme. The data analysis reveals that there are ethical challenges resulting from a complex religo-cultural understanding of the role and status of women, their autonomy, their ability to consent for participation in research and the types of research in which they are accepted or rejected by RECs in such contexts. In both countries participants spoke extensively about the nature of their "male dominant" context and how this backdrop may impact healthcare research.

> Culturally, Iran society [is] a male dominant society, as [are] many other societies in the region. But, as you may experience ... in your stay in Iran, actually, you will see that the situation has completely changed now. But, there are some default practices in the medical sector ... that, for example, are not written policies. For example, when a woman goes to a hospital for something or for research, they may ask for husband's consent, and the next level it is not official.
>
> (Iran Interview 1, Researcher, REC member, guideline developer)

> Women are certainly underrepresented on the committees. Underrepresented, which pains me greatly. We have tried to do things about that, but one of the things is that we push and shove to some degree, but the chair of the committee has a lot of say about who are the members of the committee. And who talks. By the time you've got your ... officer, [the person] isn't necessarily, but will probably be, male. The *penghulu* (chief) is always male. The head of village is always male. You've already got committees that are stacked in a

particular way with respect to gender. We ha[ve] been insistent that the gender balance [be] redress[ed] to some extent, but it's pretty weighted.

(Malaysia Interview 38, participant 38a, researcher, REC member)

This chapter[1] presents the data analysis of participants' experiences of enrolling female participants, the issue of co-consent and the ethical challenges of conducting research relating to women's health and, in particular, intimate and domestic partner violence, and women's sexual health and sexual experience. Islamic ethico-legal debates relating to *Wilayah* (guardianship), *Qiwammah* (authority), *Ta'ah* (obedience) and *Nushuz* (disobedience) will be explained in relation to women's participation in research.

The role and status of women and the appropriation of Islamic normative texts in biomedical research ethics

The data analysis indicates that the question of women's autonomy, how they are enrolled into research and how consent is obtained is an ethical dilemma for researchers. For Muslim researchers, some of the respondents explained that they found it difficult to balance their professional training of consenting the women individually with their religious and cultural beliefs about respecting the views and objections of spouses. For non-Muslim researchers, they also were unsure of how to reconcile Muslim women's own views for wanting to consult their husbands whilst trying to ensure the women themselves were sufficiently informed of the study and were able to independently enrol. There were other researchers who either did not face such challenges or felt that religious and/or cultural views on the role and status of women are unwelcome in the context of research, as they may prevent or add additional barriers to the participation of women in research. This chapter presents an analysis of some of these practical challenges and views.

Autonomy and consent of Muslim female research participants

The research ethics guidelines in Malaysia and Iran do not mention any religious or cultural consideration of co-consent (where the husband/male guardian is consented alongside the female participant) or permission (where the researcher and/or female participant are required to seek the husband/male guardian's permission). During the interviews and data analysis, however, it became clear that, despite the guidelines not including such clauses, researchers and REC members did consider the contribution from the husband, guardian and/or family as being pertinent when considering research relating to women's health and/or enrolling

---

1 Thank you to World Scientific Publishing for permission to reproduce in this chapter parts of the text from M. Suleman. (2017). Biomedical research ethics in the Islamic context: Reflections on and challenges for Islamic bioethics. In A. Bagheri & K. Alali (Eds.). *Islamic bioethics: Current issues and challenges* (pp. 197–228). (Vol. 2). Singapore: World Scientific Publishing.

women into trials. The data analysis reveals that, although very few respondents were aware of the IOMS (Islamic Organisation of Medical Sciences)[2] guidelines or other literature on the subject of Muslim women's consent (see Chapter 2), many did consider the so-called "religious" or "cultural" role of women and men as an important aspect of their enrolment procedure and cited either the *Qur'an* or sayings of the Prophet Muhammad to explain their viewpoint. For example, one of the participants in Malaysia explained:

RESEARCHER/REC MEMBER/GUIDELINE DEVELOPER: For example, informed consent. If you were to go strict with the Islamic paradigm, the wife has got to get the permission of the husband. That's the Islamic concept. And it may involve a piece of research – of course, research is something else, because we did not know the answer. For example, contraception. If you['ve] got a husband who's irresponsible, who wants lots of children every year, but not caring about the welfare of the wife – and the wife actually said, "I want a rest. I want to use contraception," and the husband said, "No," and the doctor has been approached – in our hospital we have a *Shariah* panel, we decide that yes, the wife can proceed without the husband's permission. That is a service. But, research is different, because we are talking about something unknown. But, if the husband really said, "No," and without understanding what [it]'s all about, in the Islamic paradigm, the wife has to follow the husband. For research, I don't mind [using this paradigm], but for something that is established, medical fact, our ruling or our stand in the hospital is that the wife can actually forego the husband's objection.

INTERVIEWER: Can I just ask you a couple of questions about that? First of all, what do you mean when you say, "The wife needs the husband's consent?" Could you explain that?

RESEARCHER/REC MEMBER/GUIDELINE DEVELOPER: It stems from the verse of the *Qur'an* that "Men are the protectors and maintainers of women", although this has been interpreted in many different ways. I know that in the Islamic household, the buck stops with the husband. He's the responsible person. Even if you want to go out of the house, you have to ask permission.

(Malaysia Interview 21, Researcher, REC member, guideline developer)

This interviewee presented his experience and understanding of Islam where the husband is considered the "protector" of the wife and is, therefore, given overall responsibility within a marital relationship. He did, however, explain that in instances where a medical intervention is considered of benefit to the wife, the *Shariah* panel within the hospital could override the husband's view in order to protect the rights of the woman. According to his view, as medical research is exploratory, and unless it is viewed to be of benefit to the participant's life, a husband is considered to have the right to be asked and then to be able to refuse

---

2   Please see Chapter 2 about the IOMS biomedical research ethics guidelines, which are considered an "Islamic" adaptation of the CIOMS guidelines.

her participation. This senior researcher further explained that, although he might personally disagree with the husband's view, he felt obligated to respect this "religio-cultural" dimension of authority within a marital relationship. He explained that a husband's ability to influence or deter his wife from carrying out an altruistic act might not be something he would agree with, but he would need to respect it. The researcher also reflected on a very important consideration, which is that the verse of the *Qur'an* he relies upon for developing and maintaining such an understanding of gender roles, and subsequently his responsibility in such contexts, "has been interpreted in many different ways." Although this may apply to many other ethical issues, here an analysis of the differing interpretations and related participants' views regarding women's health research will be explored.

In Malaysia, respondents explained that, despite such views about their deferring authority to husbands or male guardians in the enrolment of women in research, the guidelines do not stipulate a requirement for consulting the husband, nor do they emphasise clearly that such a consideration is unnecessary. One of the guideline developers explained that the guidelines were deliberately silent on the issue to allow researchers, participants and their families to decide for themselves. Also, the data analysis suggests that, as Malaysia is multicultural and multi-ethnic and has a national strategic interest in attracting overseas researchers and funders, the guidelines that were developed were kept non-specific.

In Iran, by contrast, one the participants explained that the issue of female consent was systematically considered when drafting the research ethics guidelines and involved formal consultation with scholars:

> As you know, in Islamic societies it's been accepted that if a lady wants to go out of her house, she should have, somehow, her husband's ... it's hard to put in [an] English word. ... I'm hesitant to use "approve", but I would like to say ... to inform her husband that she's going to go out of the house today to visit her mom, for example, [or] to do shopping. The same question was, if a female lady, if a female Muslim, is participating in a clinical research [in] which the research protocol would ask her or requires her to go to do several lab tests or physical exams, then in this case, is that okay if a female Muslim go [es] out of her house for a clinical research which her husband does not know [about]? That was the question.
> (Iran Interview 15, Researcher, REC member, guideline developer)

The data show that consultation in Iran resulted in a consensus that recommends that for non-therapeutic research, which may affect the family, both the husband and wife ought to be consulted. When researchers were asked about how this guidance works in practice, however, many explained that in Iran the consideration of consulting the spouse is understood to be the husband.

Many participants in Malaysia and Iran explained that the husband's view would be necessary if the wife's participation affected the marriage. The analysis shows that these concerns include:

- Excessive time spent away from home (away from children, household commitments)
- Accepting researchers into the home. This was considered problematic, as the house in Muslim families in Malaysia and Iran is often owned by the husband, and there may be concerns about *fitnah* (temptation) if the wife was seen to be accepting male visitors without the husband's knowledge. The analysis shows that some participants cited the authentic narration of the Prophet Muhammad where he advised that a wife should not accept visitors without her husband's permission (*Sahih Bukhari*, Book 18, *Hadith* 1750).
- If the research had the potential to affect the wife's fertility/sexual function
- If the potential participant was pregnant
- If the research concerned medical interventions that require the husband's permission, e.g., abortion, contraception, sterilisation
- If the wife or participant herself considered the husband's or male guardian's permission necessary

It is important to mention here that the data suggest that in both Malaysia and Iran, participants (both male and female) referenced this notion that a husband's permission is necessary for a wife to leave her house. Such a stipulation, however, is not made in the *Qur'an* nor in the six books of authentic sayings of the Prophet Muhammad. There are, however, references to less authentic narrations of the Prophet,[3] and the application of these in different geographical and cultural contexts will be explored in the next section.

When I asked the above participant in Iran how the issue of marital concern and consent in research is reflected in the research ethics codes, recommendations and training, he explained:

> Our recommendation was that if a research protocol would be one of those type[s] of research which we mentioned, then the ethics committee would be more concerned about informed consent, and the recommendation was that researchers would have to invite spouses and explain about the research, the methodology of research, and all these things to get their consent together, but not necessarily having two signatures for the informed consent form.
>
> (Iran Interview 15, Researcher, REC member, guideline developer)

Although the enforcement of such a recommendation may be challenging and variable, it is important to note, again, the difference in approaches between Malaysia and

---

3   In *Sunan Bayhaqi*, no. 14490, "*Ibn 'Umar* reports from the Prophet that once a lady came to the Prophet and asked him about the rights of a husband on his wife. He replied: ... she should not leave his house without his permission" (Saleem, S. (2010). *Islam and women: Misconceptions and misperceptions* (pp. 30–1). Islamic Books. https://books.google.co.uk/ books?id=E0edPU-ys7kC&pg=PA31&lpg=PA31&dq=Sunan+Bayhaqi,+No:+14490&sou rce=bl&ots=4hc56-H5RM&sig=_Hp6ijT4qSMoB5Gc4MU2oROCjIY&hl=en&sa=X&ve d=0ahUKEwjCqcqwwdvTAhVlC8AKHdY_AFwQ6AEIQjAF#v=onepage&q=Sunan%20 Bayhaqi%2C%20No%3A%2014490&f=false (Last accessed 6 May 2017)).

Iran. As there is a centralised consideration of Islamic values in Iran, the guideline developers considered it necessary to initiate a consultation on the issue of female consent, and they arrived at a conclusion that was considered acceptable according to the international expectations of ethical standards as well as the local religious considerations. In Malaysia, by contrast, although some researchers also expressed a similar concern for the family rather than a strict distinction between a man and a woman's consent, there were researchers who had experienced uncertainty. They stated that in situations where they had attempted to enrol a woman into a trial and the husband disagreed, they did not pursue her enrolment. The reasons they offered were that they considered it necessary for the husband to agree because:

- They personally consider it a religious stipulation that the husband's decision was final;
- They worried that the husband would legally contest if there was an adverse event; or
- They did not want to create marital disharmony, as this would then be considered a harm of the research.

Participants in Iran also expressed reluctance to enrol women into trials if they suspected that the husband would disagree, despite Islamic scholarly clarification that a husband's consent was not necessary:

We have done another research ... Most of them have this wrong belief ... they think that, as we are working in Islamic country, they have to [obtain husbands' consent], not because of that, because of the Islam ... They find their husbands very dangerous. They have to tell the husband, otherwise they might be in [a] problem. That's why they ask their consent, not the Islam, but they think that in Islam, that's approved. But, we have asked many scholars, many Islamic scholars of Iran, about if the women ... have to ask their husbands' consent or not. They said, "No."
(Iran Interview 13, Researcher, REC member, guideline developer)

Another senior researcher explained how as a REC they were unable to approve research that was being conducted in a "very conservative state" in Malaysia, as there were ethical concerns about the enrolment of women:

The question that we put to the researcher is that this was being done in east Malaysia, in a very conservative state in Malaysia. The questions that we ask [ed] in that setting: Do we need to get the consent from the husband? Who actually makes the decisions for the woman? Can she make it herself? Do we need her husband, or do we need her father to be around? Who actually has the consent? We couldn't decide on that. You see, if I tell you the truth, the research did not take place because there [were] ethical issues, because we couldn't resolve these issues.
(Malaysia Interview 17, Researcher, REC member, guideline developer)

The data analysis also shows that there were other researchers in Malaysia and Iran, many of whom were women, who contested the co-consent view and considered that the guidelines ought to be followed as they had been written. They thought that the issue of co-consent was cultural and had been religiously endorsed through particular interpretations of the Islamic normative sources. So, the data suggest that, although many of the researchers considered an approach where they were keen to accommodate a woman's belief or concern for consulting her husband, the husband's expression of a strong opinion or the researcher's own belief that it was appropriate to allow time for husband or family consultation, there were some researchers and REC members who were critical of this approach. They disagreed with this view of women's autonomy. Many expressed frustration at there being a lack of adherence to guidelines. The data analysis shows that in Malaysia, the issue of co-consent or deferral to the husband was not primarily a religious concern, as it was encountered with non-Muslim participants also. Participants in Malaysia and Iran explained that this was due to cultural influence, and this cultural impression of the role and status of women had permeated into a religious narrative, the latter accentuating the former.

> I think that some people have idea about Islam and generalize this idea to all Muslims, all Muslim countries or all people, but we easily know that this is not what Islam says.
> (Iran Interview 1, Researcher, REC member, guideline developer)

> I think [it is] a cultural problem we have to respect. It's not [an] Islamic problem.
> (Iran Interview 13, Researcher, REC member, guideline developer)

> I think, yeah, [it is] so important to point all this out to the researcher ... Yes, there are going to be differences of opinion; and people bring with them their cultural understanding or lack of understanding of different things; and you, too, have all [of] this; but I think there are standards, and there are clear guidelines, and we as medical professionals, researchers should stick to those.
> (Malaysia Interview 29, Researcher, REC member, guideline developer)

Understanding autonomy and the concepts of Wilayah, Qiwamah, Ta'ah and Nushuz

This section will review the data analysis of the *Quranic* concepts of *Wilayah* (guardianship of men over women), *Qiwamah* (a degree of strength/authority that is afforded to men over women), *Ta'ah* (obedience) and *Nushuz* (disobedience) in relation to biomedical research ethics. The above section highlights that during the discussions with participants about the enrolment of female participants into trials, the religious and cultural impressions of the role of men and women became important. The data analysis shows that, in terms of the religious context, participants offered verses of the *Qur'an* or *Hadith* as explanations for their views. As these references were expressed by participants as being important, it became clear during the interviews that a deeper analysis of these views and interpretations was necessary in order to understand whether it was the Islamic normative sources that were informing such views, or if cultural influences were resulting in particular interpretations of these sources, or a combination of the two. One of the participants in Iran expressed very strong views about consent and autonomy in Muslim societies, and what he articulated as an Islamic perspective rooted in the normative sources of Islam:

INTERVIEWER: Are there any particular issues that involve faith or an Islamic consideration?

RESEARCHER/REC MEMBER: One of the question[s] is feminism. I think it seems ... mainstream ... in Western countries ... Feminism is against the Islamic thought. In Islam we study the *Qur'an*. No feminism. No manism or other. The *Qur'an* says "Whosoever doeth right, whether male or female, and is a believer..." [in Arabic]. Men and women have different bod[ies], but their souls are the same. It's the same. That aspect of [a] human being that referred to God and the soul, the spirit – there is no man, no woman. Feminism focused on this. Research about family and women in Western countr[ies] take[s] impression of feminism.

(Iran Interview 11, Researcher, REC member)

He explained, as other respondents indicated, that the Islamic tradition does not focus on the individual, it focuses on the relationship with God. Decision-making also is not focused on the individual, but the family. He further explained that when two people, a man and a woman, come together to create a family, their roles and their autonomy are different to when they are single. He explained that in Islam the role of the family is more important than the individuals within it. However, the family itself requires a lead:

RESEARCHER/REC MEMBER: When a woman and when a man are separated, they then come together and create a family. They [each] have [a] different job and different position in [the] family. We say from Prophet Mohammed: "If you are traveling, and you are only three person, one of you must be superior." Social job. Not superiority [of] spirit and soul. Social job. In this area and this workplace, you are superior. A woman [may be] superior of man in his job, but in family, because many aspect[s] of physiology of man and woman, I think, it seems that Islam give[s] man a superiority for management of family. It [does] not mean that man is better than woman. The *Qur'an* says "Whosoever doeth right, whether male or female, and is a believer..." [in Arabic].

INTERVIEWER: Would you then say the autonomy of a man and a woman is different?

RESEARCHER/REC MEMBER: Autonomy of man and woman, unmarried, is different [from] autonomy of man and woman that [are] married. Autonomy of mine, before I married my wife, is different to after I was married. I have lower autonomy after I got married. My autonomy is lower because I accept my job in my family. I have commitment to my wife. My wife [is the] same to me.

(Iran Interview 11, Researcher, REC member)

The data suggest that this characterisation of autonomy is distinct to the description in, for example, Beauchamp and Childress's (2001) seminal work on biomedical ethics (pp. 57–103). Although the analysis and the participant's description seem to point to both men and women having equal responsibility and freedom to serve the needs of their family, the quote highlights that, according to the respondent's interpretation of the *Qur'an*, the man has been given "superiority" and, therefore, may exercise the power to set the agenda for what is in the family's best interests.

Other participants described problems with such a view, which relies on the supposition that the man can decide what these "best interests" are without unduly placing his needs above the needs of his wife and family. Respondents explained that there may be conflicts of interest, which may cause problems, including the wife's inability to act altruistically. Her husband may, for example, intervene and prevent her enrolment, arguing for her safety. However, he may be, in fact, more concerned for his own convenience, such as ensuring he does not have to unduly take on more responsibility for the children or housework. Researchers explained that disentangling such motivations might be incredibly complex and unachievable.

Others also contested the above interpretation of *Wilayah* (guardianship) and *Qiwamah* (authority):

I'm completely against it, because the meaning of "*Qawwamun*" does not mean that men should protect their women. It does not mean that. It reprises some aspects of the priority of men to women, but just in one verse of the *Qur'an*, not in the other verses of the *Qur'an*. I think that men and women are completely equal, and they have equal rights. Nobody can make decisions for women. Women should make their decisions and should control their autonomy by [themselves], and their husbands cannot influence their autonomy. I consider the women's autonomy as absolute, as well. It is not relative ... I think they misuse the *Qur'an*. They use the *Qur'an*, but they want it to provide facts for their beliefs from the *Qur'an*. But it is not a good way to use the *Qur'an* – [to the detriment of] our beliefs. It is bizarre utilization of the *Qur'an*. It is not fair, I think.

(Iran Interview 12, Researcher, REC member)

Actually, I think it is unreasonable to ask the husband to sign a consent form on behalf of his wife or in addition to the consent of his wife. I think it is unreasonable and unethical. I think because the woman is a human being, and she is free to take part in the study or not ... I think we can interpret the Islam whatever we want, and this is the main problem in our world. That in Saudi Arabia they interpret the *Qur'an* and Islam, and here it is different ... I think the right of the subject is the basic part of our research. It has nothing to do with any religion like Islam, because if we think about these issues like a pyramid, the base is human rights. We are talking about humans, and they have some rights regardless of their religion or their beliefs. Because I think [in] the first instance people are human, then they are Iranian and then they are Muslim. I think we need to address this.

(Iran Interview 6, Researcher, REC member)

Some of the participants stressed the importance of looking at different environments to understand why particular interpretations of Islam and the scriptural sources are taken. Several participants in Iran mentioned that the Iranian understanding of the role and status of women was distinct to that in other parts of the Muslim world, particularly the Arab states. One author, who studied Muslim family law in Arab countries, analysed what is commonly considered to be "patriarchal religiously-justified laws in Muslim countries" (Al-Hibri, 1997, p. 2). Her study looked at the personal status codes of Egypt, Algeria, Morocco, Tunisia, Syria, Jordan and Kuwait. All of these countries, until recently, "listed or implied a duty of obedience (*ta'ah*) by the wife" (Al-Hibri, 1997, p. 11). Recent political changes in Tunisia have brought family law reforms that replaced the "obedience" clause with the man simply being described as the head of the family (Al-Hibri, 1997, p. 11). These codes are important, as they specify that obedience includes a wife's inability to leave the husband's house without his permission. If she were to leave without permission, she would be deemed sinful, disobedient (*nushuz*) and no longer eligible for financial support (Al-Hibri, 1997, p. 12). Such constructions of Islamic law and interpretations of scripture, though formed in Arab states, have influenced the learning and understanding in countries like Malaysia and Iran. Although women occupy the highest positions in office in both of these countries, there is a lack of clarity about what the "Islamic" understanding is in relation to the role and status of women. Many of the participants, including scholars, explained that the verses mentioning *Wilayah, Qiwwamah, ta'ah* and *Nushuz* were commonly interpreted and applied in isolation of the broader message of the *Qur'an*, which emphasises equality between men and women:

Because the Muslims think their wives are their possession[s], I don't think so and so, because I don't think ... she, [the] wife, is independent to do the thing [that] is good for her or what is bad for her. She doesn't need to ask the permission from her husband in this case, because this, as I said, this is a type of Muslim who think[s] that their wife [is] their possession. Because of the possession, the wife cannot do anything without the permission from the husband. This is a very orthodox view of Muslim in the sense.

(Malaysia Interview 27, Islamic scholar, REC member)

The scholar explained that Islam and its ability to influence behaviour and wield political or social power is used to enforce or accentuate a particular culture. As explained in Chapter 1, Islamic jurisprudence enables the use of culture or *Urf* to set religious norms and individual reasoning or *ijtihad* [4] by scholars to emphasise particular values and principles. Some of the participants explained that they disagreed with such a system of interpretation. One scholar explained that such interpretations are as a result of "male-dominated" or patriarchal interpretations of the *Qur'an*, where Islamic scholarship, especially the translation and interpretation of the *Qur'an*, has been led by male scholars:

> I don't agree to that kind of interpretation, because for me, Islam takes responsibility on [an] individual basis ... This also proves that as a wife, she does not have to rely solely on her husband ... Yeah, because the *Mufasirun* (commentators on the *Qur'an*) are Muslim men [chuckles]. *Mufasirun* are mostly Muslim men. They think about themselves, not about the welfare of the spouses, in my understanding of those *Mufasirun*. They look from their point of view ... This is a very sad story of a Muslim. This is how people understand some *Quranic* text[s] for their own sake, not for the sake of others. They think that they are truly correct in understanding, and those who are different from them [are] wrong.
>
> (Malaysia Interview 27, Islamic scholar, REC member)

The scholar expressed the view and concern of many of the participants in Malaysia and Iran, who considered it necessary to constantly survey the laws of Islam and re-examine religious interpretation and jurisprudence to ensure the rights of women and men and the interests of society are met given the evolving local and global contexts and cultures. Participants' differing views, however, indicate a complex interplay of culture and religion through the interpretation and application of religious texts.

In light of the data analysis illustrating participants' views relating to the sensitivity of *Quranic* interpretation, it is important to briefly consider the factors that influence *Quranic* interpretation. Authors who have written on this subject state that there are at least four factors to consider (Von Denffer, 1983, pp. 41–2):

• What is said within the text, and whether the text itself can be an explanation
• Consideration of a verse/text within the whole revelation and the whole period of revelation
• When the text itself is open, it is important to consider the cultural projection or the environment of revelation, including the tradition of the Prophet Muhammad
• The interpretation of the text through the tradition of scholars, e.g., each of the four/five schools of Islamic law may have their own rules of *Quranic* interpretation

4 Please see Chapters 1 and 3 for more information about the process of *ijtihad*.

Thus far, for the interpretation of the word "*qawwamun*", the "superiority" of men over women has been most commonly used, followed by "having authority over". Less common interpretations include "take care of" or "are responsible for" (Abou Bakr, 2015, pp. 44–62). Some authors have even suggested that the term could mean that men are the "servants" of women (El Fadl, 2014, p. 210). The last two interpretations emphasise that the man has the duty to take care of the family, and the woman has the right not to work and be looked after. Many participants, however, shared the former and not the latter interpretations.

My data analysis shows that researchers and REC members, particularly women,[5] are seeking to challenge the former interpretations and traditional gender roles that they think may impact women's ability to access healthcare and participate in biomedical research. The respondents explained, as seen in the quotes above, that they disagree with such interpretations of the term *qawwamun* and prefer a more contemporary understanding of gender roles within the family and wider society. They also explained that the verse mentioning *qawwamun* ought to be considered alongside the other verses of the *Qur'an* that emphasise equality between women and men, and women ought to decide for themselves whether or not they want to enrol in research studies. Their views reflect the science of *Quranic* interpretation, a summary of which is listed above, which stipulates the need for interpreting each verse in light of the entire text.

The data show that there are differing views. Some participants considered the Islamic understanding of autonomy to be distinct, and the role of the husband/ male guardian was vital to their deliberations around autonomy and consent in the context of biomedical research. Such differing views also prevailed between researchers and their participants as well as the wider public.

Challenges relating to women's health and wellbeing

From the above analysis of the perspectives of researchers, REC members, guideline developers and scholars in my interviews, it is evident that the interpretation of religious scripture and the role of culture in determining the role and status of women are contested. Some participants explained that an important ethical consideration is that women are often marginalised in certain, especially rural, communities and may not access healthcare and health research. They also described how their research is impacted when they conduct studies in communities where women are required to seek permission to leave the house and/or fulfil particular roles within the family. An analysis of their experiences highlights key emerging ethical issues and practical challenges relating to the role and status of women and how certain cultural views and practices are reinforced by particular scriptural interpretations. The analysis shows that the interaction between culture and religious scriptural interpretation raises ethical tensions and challenges for researchers,

---

5   See quotes from female participants in this study, such as Iran participants 6, 12 and 13 and Malaysia participants 25, 28 and 29.

particularly when investigating domestic and intimate partner violence and the sexual health and sexual experience of women.

Intimate and domestic partner violence

The World Health Organization (WHO) has reported that "violence against women by an intimate partner is a major contributor to the ill-health of women" (Garcia-Moreno et al., 2006, p. vi). Views expressed by participants revealed that research on intimate and domestic partner violence was challenging in Muslim contexts, beyond issues of privacy, confidentiality, safety and participant vulnerability, which have been described previously by other studies (Ellsberg et al., 2001). The data analysis shows that what is considered domestic violence is contextually dependent. Some participants explained that due to the acceptance of "*wilayah*" in Muslim households, where the man is considered the "guardian" or "superior", there is a different understanding of "domestic violence". Of course, contextual adaptations and translations of such terms are necessary. However, from some of the participants' views, it was apparent that they were reluctant to conduct or approve such research. One of the female researchers in Iran explained that such concerns had little to do with Islam or scriptural interpretation, and they had more to do with cultural influences and husbands feeling threatened by such research. She explained:

> For example, in our country, based on our cultural issues, it's very difficult to ask women about domestic violence ... [It] may [cause] them problem[s] in their home, and their husbands make it difficult to do that research, too, and they make complaint[s] about that research ... [Groups that research women's views and experiences may] have made a focus group, which means women [talk] about their right[s] in [their] family, and after that, women feel very regret[ful]. Those focus group[s] influence them to find that they're not satisfied [in] their lives, and that makes their families problem[atic] ... Their husbands get frustrated and complain about that research, "You're not allowed to involve our wives in this research. You're not allowed to ask them to give you their experience[s] of ... domestic violence, their rights, and what kind of life they wish to have." That's, I think, a cultural problem we have to respect. It's not [an] Islamic problem ... and they couldn't continue that research ... those who are governing that province say, "Stop that research ... you're not allowed to do this research in our province because of the cultural issues we have. You're not allowed."
>
> (Iran Interview 13, Researcher, REC member, guideline developer)

There was an appreciable sensitivity about such research, as the men felt threatened that their wives would demand a different relationship and different freedoms. Although, in Iran there are differing views about a wife's ability to freely leave her home, decide who she meets and determine who she invites into the home, there is an underlying concern regarding conducting such research.

The WHO study on intimate partner violence stated that it is particularly diffi-cult to study and respond effectively to such violence, as many women and socie-ties accept such violence as "normal". When researchers were asked about such concerns, they explained that one particular verse of the *Qur'an* (*The Holy Qur'an,* Chapter 4, verse 34) has been interpreted, accepted and applied within contexts in which they work to not only justify such violence, but it has caused Muslim women to feel that they must accept such treatment as being within the fold of Islam, and they are deserving of such violence because of their own behaviour:

> When you talk about values, for example, it's very difficult for people, for survivors of domestic violence, to actually just disconnect with their husband [s] because they think that religion gives a certain interpretation about men and wives' relationships. Now, how do you tell a woman, a survivor, for example, about obedience? This is critical values when you talk about intimate kind of violence in a Muslim culture. ... I realise this is not just Muslim cul-ture, but in any faith community, in fact, because, in my studies, it comes up like 30 percent are Christians, 30 percent are Hindus and 30 percent are Muslim. They just come up, naturally.
>
> When you talk about obedience, for example, most of these religions, most of these believers of these religion, I'll put it that way, believe that women must obey their husbands, but they stop short there. When you want to engage them on this dialogue about what obedience is all about, you're really trying to intrude into their faiths sometimes, because you're trying to get them to have this dialogue with you. Sometimes, I wonder whether that is right to do. But, at the same time, I also wonder what would happen if you don't do [it]. Will they just get stuck with that knowledge? Shouldn't we then engage them with this dialogue about the whole idea of obedience? As a researcher, if you know you just don't want to engage them in this dialogue, then just leave them and go on with your research, continue to finish up your research. Who will then support them to continue with this dialogue, this religious dialogue that you have started with them? That is important, isn't it? Do we start this dialogue with them or not? If I don't do it, at the back of my mind, as a believer, ... I want to give them information. Who can give this information, and what kind of information that they should have so that they can process this whole idea about this rules that they have in mind about obedience so that they can be really knowledgeable, so that they can make the right decision?
>
> (Malaysia Interview 25, Researcher, REC member)

The researcher's experience reveals a deep ethical challenge. As a Muslim herself, she feels it is important to represent her faith, but she is concerned about the sci-entific requirements of the study and the ethical and welfare implications of her intervention. She is also concerned about her ethical obligation to simply respect the women's views about their marital relationships, whilst balancing her spiritual concern for sharing her own beliefs and understanding of the religion. How personal faith interacts with researchers' concerns about their professional obligations will be explored more in Chapter 6. However, it is important to point out here the emphasis on a trend discovered in her research, whereby many religions, not only Islam, have particular ideas about "obedience" of the wife within marriage.

One of the scholars in Malaysia expressed a deep concern about such scriptural interpretations, and the extent to which such interpretations are being politicised. He explained that a non-government organisation (NGO), which had been working hard to lobby for women's rights, had a religious edict (*fatwah*) issued against them, causing their work to be put under scrutiny. He also explained that in Malaysia there is a specific law that has been issued to protect women, however, differing interpretations of the aforementioned *Quranic* verse have meant that women themselves are unable to challenge their circumstances. Rather, they feel it is their religious obligation to accept the status quo:

> The woman are very afraid of going against her husbands' wishes, desires or whatever ... We have laws in Malaysia to protect women, but they don't go and report, because they say that if she reports her problem, the family will get shamed or something like that. This is also a type of misleading teaching that is making Muslim people suffer, especially women in this condition. They are suffering. [First,] for religious sake, for example, as she was told, and she accepted that. Second, it's shameful to the family. Third, if the wife does not have any job to support her for economy's sake. She is there. These are among the reasons that [is] what happened, and still happens. I think she has to go to NGOs. This is also a problem in Malaysia. Do you know about Sisters in Islam in Malaysia? The Sisters in Islam was accused by the mufti of Selangor, the state ... mufti of Selangor [of] practicing or, I don't know, religious pluralism and secularism.
>
> (Malaysia Interview 27, Islamic scholar, REC member)

His experience highlights some key challenges when trying to conduct research on intimate and domestic partner violence. He points out that the so-called religious objection to the promotion of women's rights is on the basis that such views are "unIslamic" or "secular", and that such secularisation ought to be challenged. He also suggests that such views exist and remain within societies not because of the religion per se, but because of women's lack of economic freedom.

The data analysis also shows that the interpretation of the *Quranic* verse, Chapter 4, verse 34, is contested, and Islamic scholars in Malaysia and Iran do not consider the verse as granting permission for husbands to hit their wives. One of the Islamic scholars explained that the word "*darabah*" does not mean "to hit"; rather, it means to "move away". The data analysis also shows that the interpretation suggesting that men can hit their wives has been prevalent and accepted by many women, particularly in rural areas, as being a "religious" instruction. Recent developments in Islamic scholarship and the literature on the issue of "wife beating", particularly from the perspective of Muslim female scholars, will be discussed in Chapter 7.

Women's sexual health and sexual experience

Challenges regarding the study of women's health were also appreciable in researchers' accounts of trying to investigate women's sexual health and sexual experience. One researcher explained that the barrier to her research was not simply underlying religious-based assumptions of male authority, where husbands prevented or stopped the research; she said the female participants considered it a religious responsibility to keep what is between the husband and wife private. She also explained that most Muslim women she spoke to tend to be highly religious and would not want to act in contradiction to their faith. The researcher expressed emotional difficulty when explaining the barriers she encountered when trying to conduct research on sexual violence within marriage, women's sexual experiences and their sexual health. She considered that there is a great need for such research and felt unsupported by her colleagues and community:

> I think it's based on our education, because we were being told what happened in the bedroom is private. You are not supposed to share it with anybody. When I spoke to some of the women, although they agreed to discuss with me, they [said] specific issues in relation to sexuality. They said they cannot talk about it ... [they said] it's a sin to talk about your personal issues to do with your husband ... At the moment in Malaysia, issues relating to sexuality in women [are] actually on the rise. Nobody is actually doing research out there that actually looks into why women are becoming victims. I see that these women, they're more obeying. I'm a wife. I have to obey my husband. It doesn't really matter whether my experience sexually, whether it's satisfied a lot. It doesn't matter. The important thing is I obey my husband. I'm a good housewife. I have to fulfil my husband's needs. There is the current situation in Malaysia. I believe that this issue was never discussed openly. When you do research in sexuality, people will say, "Why do you want to do research?" Even the first time when I started, when I proposed, people are saying, "Why do you want to do it with women? Women have to obey their husband." Even doctors may speak to them saying, "No. I don't think you should do research on this."
>
> (Malaysia Interview 28, Researcher)

The researcher's experience and the data analysis highlight what some authors have considered to be religious-based understandings of male authority and their underlying assumptions (Mir-Hosseini et al., 2015, pp. 1–10). The concept of Muslim women having to be obedient and sexually available to their husbands has been contested (Mir-Hosseini, 2015, p. 13–40), yet authors argue that such gender roles remain entrenched, particularly in more rural communities (Garcia-Moreno et al., 2006). The data also highlight ethical concerns researchers experience around not only barriers to carrying out such research, but also the lack of support and moral anxiety in these contexts, with beliefs or values that are at odds with their research community, colleagues and potential participants. These ethical concerns will be explored further in Chapter 7.

Conclusions

In summary, the data analysis shows firstly, that there are ethical challenges resulting from a complex religio-cultural understanding of the role and status of women, their autonomy and ability to consent for participation in research and also the types of research that are accepted or rejected by RECs in such contexts. Participants' views also indicate a complex interplay of culture and religion through the interpretation and application of religious texts. In both countries, at the level of researchers and RECs, the data show that there is a variation in understanding what ought to be done when enrolling women in research and the types of studies that can be undertaken involving women's health.

Secondly, it also emerged from the data that the notion of autonomy understood by some researchers in Malaysia and Iran is different to that understood in the "Western" secular construct. The data analysis suggests that the Islamic tradition does not focus on the individual, but on their relationship with God. Decision-making also is not focused on the individual, but the family. Thirdly, such understandings of autonomy come up against notions of *Wilayah, Qiwammah, Ta'ah* and *Nushuz*. The analysis shows that differing interpretations of the latter terms raise ethical tensions and challenges for researchers, particularly when investigating domestic and intimate partner violence and the sexual health and sexual experience of women.

Bibliography

Abou Bakr, O. (2015). The interpretative legacy of Qiwamah as an exegetical construct. In Z. Mir-Hosseini, M.Al-Sharmani & J. Rumminger (Eds.). *Men in charge?: Rethinking authority in Muslim legal tradition* (pp. 44–62). London: Oneworld Publications.

Al-Hibri, A. Y. (1997). Islam, law and custom: Redefining Muslim women's rights. *American University Journal of International Law and Policy*, 12(1), 1. http://scholarship.richmond.edu/cgi/viewcontent.cgi?article=1157&context=law-faculty-publications (Last accessed 19 August 2016).

Beauchamp, T. L. & Childress, J. F. (2001). *Principles of biomedical ethics*. New York: Oxford University Press.

El Fadl, K. A. (2014). *Speaking in God's name: Islamic law, authority and women*. Oxford: Oneworld Publications.

Ellsberg, M., Heise, L., Pena, R., Agurto, S. & Winkvist, A. (2001). Researching domestic violence against women: Methodological and ethical considerations. *Stud Fam Plann*, 32(1), 1–16.

Garcia-Moreno, C., Jansen, H. A., Ellsberg, M., Heise, L. & Watts, C. H. (2006). Prevalence of intimate partner violence: Findings from the WHO multi-country study on women's health and domestic violence. *The Lancet*, 368(9543), 1260–1269.

Mir-Hosseini, Z. (2015). Muslim legal tradition and the challenge of gender equality. In Z. Mir-Hosseini, M.Al-Sharmani & J. Rumminger (Eds.). *Men in charge?: Rethinking authority in Muslim legal tradition* (pp. 13–40). London: Oneworld Publications.

Mir-Hosseini, Z., Al-Sharmani, M. & Rumminger, J. (Eds.). (2015). *Men in charge?: Rethinking authority in Muslim legal tradition*. London: Oneworld Publications.

Sahih Bukahri. Book 18, Hadith 1750. http://sunnah.com/riyadussaliheen/18/240 (Last accessed 19 August 2016).

Saleem, S. (2010). *Islam and women: Misconceptions and misperceptions.* Islamic Books.

Suleman M. (2016). Contributions and ambiguities in Islamic research ethics and research conducted in Muslim contexts: I – A thematic review of the literature. *Journal of Health and Culture* 1 (1), 46–57.

Suleman, M. (2017). Biomedical research ethics in the Islamic context. Reflections on and challenges for Islamic bioethics. In A. Bagheri & K. A. Ali (Eds.). *Islamic bioethics: Current issues and challenges* (Vol. 2, pp. 197–228). Singapore: World Scientific Publishing.

The Holy Qur'an. Chapter 4, verse 34. http://corpus.quran.com/translation.jsp?chapter=4&verse=34 (Last accessed 2 March 2016).

Von Denffer, A. (1983). *Ulum al Quran.* The Islamic Foundation.

6 Personal faith and biomedical research ethics

Encountering the moral universe of Muslim researchers

Previous chapters presented an analysis of the institutional forms of Islam that are involved in biomedical research ethics and how these institutional forms face pressures, such as those associated with HIV/AIDS. A related theme arising in my analysis of the interviews was that the individuals within these institutional forms of Islam, such as biomedical researchers, REC members, guideline developers, contextual and bridge scholars, are personally struggling with balancing different priorities and value systems, including their own faith. The data indicate that these deliberations have a very important influence in being able to consider whether and how Islam influences biomedical research ethics. Some of these deliberations will be presented in this chapter.

When faced with a practical problem, such as the need to address the HIV/AIDS epidemic or whether and how to enrol women into a research study, the analysis shows that researchers in these contexts concurrently have to consider what is recommended by physicians' codes of conduct, research ethics guidelines, global health priorities, as well as what is instructed by Islam and its formal structures together with local cultural values. This chapter presents an analysis of how participants personally deliberate over the practical problems of HIV/AIDS and researching and meeting the health needs of women, which require them to reconcile their different value systems.

What also emerges from the data is that, in addressing such practical challenges, respondents expressed a deep commitment to Islamic ethics and law, which influences their understanding of their legal and moral accountability. This personal accountability originating from participants' faith commitments adds an additional layer of complexity to the institutional forms of Islam when the latter are engaged to address the ethical challenges of global health problems like HIV/AIDS. This chapter also looks again at the cross-cutting theme of Islamic scholarly authority by analysing the experiences of biomedical researchers and REC members as not only contributors of the contextual information for *ijtihad*, but also as drivers or advocates for particular types of research through their professional obligations and understanding of the global biomedical context.

Conscientious objection, moral intuitions and beliefs about legal and moral accountability in HIV/AIDS research

The institutional forms of Islam presented in Chapter 3, in reality, comprise individuals who are expected to assess and address health research pressures and possible competing values and interests. Although previous chapters briefly included some of these deliberations, as these personal negotiations appeared to be very significant in my data analysis, it is important to present a summary here as an independent chapter.

Chapter 4 presented how global health challenges, such as HIV/AIDS, have stimulated Islam's institutional elements to engage with issues that are illegal to address the health needs of IVDUs, sex workers and MSMs. The data show how some issues, like that of approving needle exchange programmes for IVDUs, have been negotiated and approved by Islam's institutional forms. However, other issues, including researching and addressing the health needs of sex workers and MSMs, have not been addressed in the same way. The analysis in Chapter 4 suggested that this may be due to the taboo and socio-culturally unacceptable nature of these sexual practices. Further examination of the personal deliberations of respondents in this chapter offers additional insights into how researchers and REC members negotiate such practical problems and what the underlying values may be in such deliberations.

The data show that in both Malaysia and Iran, some participants expressed how they were unable to consider barrier contraception as an acceptable research intervention to assess the latter's efficacy in curtailing the spread of HIV/AIDS:

> [T]hese are very important problems, but they are not acceptable based on Islam rules, and investigation about them, from my view, is not acceptable … This relationship exists, I do not deny it, but based on our religion, they are not acceptable. Any investigation about it means that we are accepting this action, but they are not acceptable. From my view, any investigation about this problem means that we are accept[ing] it as a formal action, while they are not acceptable based on our religion.
>
> (Iran Interview 7, Researcher, REC member)

> I think it is quite against what I believe, because I believe that we need to have a … what do you call [it]? Men and women need to be in an official marriage … I don't know how to … The relationship must be official, and then, only, they can have sex or whatever, but if you say it is before that they do it, they did that, so to me it is against the religion first of all. If I really want to understand the issue, I will conduct research to understand the issue … If I really want to understand the issue, my aim is to help to reduce the numbers … My aim is that. Not really whether they wear protection. It is not that. If I ask them whether they wear protection, and then [I say], "Oh you should wear protection," meaning that I agree that you can have sex

before marriage, but you need to wear protection. Something like that. It is against my belief ... For me you cannot do it until you get married. Then, only, I can ask whether you wear protection or not. Something like that. The discussion is on the behaviour, and how we are going to prevent it.

(Malaysia Interview 12, Researcher, REC member)

There is a tension that arises. Although researchers accept that the research and health needs associated with HIV/AIDS exist, and that, professionally, they ought to be addressed, they consider that by researching these communities, they inadvertently breach their faith obligations. Such conscientious objection resembles that seen for abortion, where a health need may be recognised, however, due to a practitioner's own faith or moral commitments, they refuse to participate in a termination. The analysis also points to notions of moral and legal accountability, where researchers feel they would be culpable for supporting such illegal activities.

Other participants, however, explained that they were unable to ignore the health need and felt it was important to try to reconcile the two sources of moral thinking, personal and professional, by combining them: educating against extra-marital relations (fulfilling what they considered a religious obligation), whilst providing a temporary means of researching and curtailing the spread of the epidemic through the distribution of condoms and needles (a public health intervention).

The data analysis reveals an additional tension – public perception or cultural barriers to carrying out research on marginalised groups. One researcher explained that, although he had religious reservations about approving research on sex workers and MSMs, his concerns were also linked to the potential public outcry if such research was widely approved and conducted in Malaysia:

RESEARCHER/REC MEMBER: In terms of ... the perspective of religion ... we have never done trials like what people have done in Cambodia, for instance. HIV trials in sex workers. It has never been done in this country, so we never will challenge ... Here, many of the Muslim doctors would probably object, in the sense that you are ... encouraging prostitution, for instance, among the sex workers ... I am sure that I and my other Muslim colleagues would have raised an objection, or [we] would have become very critical about it. Because, certain things, the Muslims here share common things, like [attitudes toward] promiscuities. As you know, [they] are things [that] are very standard. They're like any other Muslim country. If you are seeing that you must give a drug [and] compare two groups of sex workers while you give [it to] them ... I don't think we would have participated, the reason being you are encouraging the whole thing.

INTERVIEWER: What are your reasons for that? What are your reasons for thinking that is a problem?

RESEARCHER/REC MEMBER: Well, the higher good, of course, is that whether [the drug] works and helps to prevent the spread of the disease. Like I said, it could be I do that. It should be maybe okay. But, at the ground level, if the public knows that we are bringing [in groups of sex workers], and some of the things that we do would encourage prostitution in the future. Because, you know, you can prevent this and, therefore, I think most of the Muslim doctors would be uncomfortable.

INTERVIEWER: Is that discomfort because of your faith, or because of that public perception?

RESEARCHER/REC MEMBER: Both, I think. For most of us, it may be faith, but the second point about perception is also very important. We don't want to be seen to be doing these, yeah.

(Malaysia Interview 6, Researcher, REC member)

His practical deliberation and that of other researchers and REC members about the issue of researching HIV/AIDS spread amongst sex workers raises questions about the complex interplay between religion and culture underlying the concerns about the acceptability of such research. The participant explained that if a drug or similar intervention could be implemented to prevent the spread of HIV/AIDS, then this would be a "higher good" according to the higher objectives of the *Shariah* (*Maqasid* – see Chapter 4). However, he explained that concerns about permitting prostitution or homosexuality and the public perception and outcry about such practices meant that researchers and REC members like him felt uncomfortable with conducting and approving such studies.

Some Muslim researchers, however, explained that they kept their individual faith obligations personal, and placed their professional responsibility as a primary practical concern:

I wear more of my doctor hat in this case, and [my] public health hat and my role is not to tell them to be a good Muslim, my role is to tell them how to protect themselves and that's it, simple. I'm not the Imam. If they want to seek spiritual guidance or whatever, then I'm not the person. If that is wrong in the eyes of God, well, I'll pay for it later on, but to me, I think we're all adults. We can make decisions right or wrong, and same with sex workers ... allowing sex workers to work as sex workers because they need to earn a living.

(Malaysia Interview 29, Researcher, REC member)

The researcher explained that she considers her relationship with Islam and the normative texts as being very important and integral to her worldview, and although she considers extramarital relations and homosexuality unlawful, she conceded that such concerns or tensions are beyond her professional obligations. As stated above, the researcher passionately explained that "if that is wrong in the eyes of God, well, I'll pay for it later on". Her statement is very powerful in that she considers her worldview and her metaphysical reality as she deliberates how she can reconcile the two. Her reference to God relates to the Islamic paradigm that many other participants emphasised in that they considered the normative sources of Islam, namely the *Qur'an* and the Prophet's *Hadith* as their ultimate source of moral guidance. Participants also explained that the *Quranic* emphasis on the belief in the oneness of God (*tawhid*) that they have chosen to ascribe to, influences their understanding of many aspects of ethico-moral thinking, such as: how should we live, what makes an action right or wrong, and how do we decide where our understanding of right and wrong comes from. As explained in previous chapters, although rational thinking is considered an important aspect of moral understanding within the Islamic tradition, as it is required not only to interpret normative scripture but to also enable a rational understanding of right and wrong, such intellectual reasoning is only one of three tools for ethico-legal decision-making. The data analysis suggests that, in addition to reason, there are two other sources of moral decision-making that Muslim researchers may engage with, which are one's intuitive nature (*fitr'a*) and revelation (*wahy*) (see Chapter 1).

The data shows that researchers who prioritise their professional obligations and, therefore, provide services for sex workers and research their health needs, consider the lifestyle choices of such groups to be independent of the care they provide. Respondents also explained that they were uncomfortable making moral judgements about how sex workers choose to earn a living given the constraints of their socio-economic reality. Many of the researchers considered a systemic management of such problems ideal, where a society could be formed where people did not have to undertake such illegal work. However, many did accept that marginalised groups exist, and they need to be researched, and health services need to be researched and designed appropriately to meet their health needs. The analysis shows that researchers' practical deliberations about such issues involves a combination of considering what God's revelation stipulates (accepting that certain activities are illegal) as well as what their reason and intuitive nature are causing them to understand (the necessity to research and meet the health needs of such groups).

The relationship between reason (*aql*), revelation (*wahy*) and one's intuitive nature (*fitr'a*), within the context of biomedical research ethics in Malaysia and Iran reveals a complex nexus of moral decision-making amongst Muslim researchers. Those who choose not to engage in research involving illicit practices not only describe a reliance on revelation, but they also talk about the need for cultivating and keeping in harmony with an Islamic moral character. Within the Islamic tradition, intuition, or *fitr'a*, is not the same as that understood within the Western tradition, where intuition has been defined as "a highly personal voice" (Ives & Dunn, 2010, p258) and "our assumptions about what is right and wrong" (Ives & Dunn, 2010, p. 259). In Islam, by contrast, intuitions are described as one's natural disposition that originates from God and is thus inclined towards good (Sachedina, 2009; Ahmed & Suleman, 2018). Reliance on one's intuitive nature for Muslim researchers, therefore, involves a deep commitment to personal moral cultivation, such that one can access the *fitr'a*. This lifelong exercise is similar to Aristotelean *phronesis* and provides an insight into the multiple moral sources that Muslim researchers may rely on, and how their decision-making may not be a predictable reflection of what is conferred through traditional Islamic authority, such as Muslim scholarly deliberations and *fatawah.* A tradition of the Prophet Muhammad (Sahih Muslim, Book 22, Hadith 133) describes what is involved in personal moral cultivation to enable access to the *fitr'a*, where he emphasises the boundary between what is lawful (*halal*) and unlawful (*haram*) as doubtful (*shubahaat*). He further explains that protecting and cultivating one's moral character (the seat of which is the heart in the Islamic tradition) requires one to refrain from the doubtful. For Muslim researchers who consider emerging biomedical research challenges like HIV/AIDs as an area where there is ongoing scholarly debate and disagreement, the data show that they thus consider the actions to address HIV/AIDs as morally doubtful. Subsequently, they choose to err on the side of remaining disengaged from such activities.

The data analysis also raises a very important issue regarding the tensions that arise in the prioritisation between professional and personal values. The above respondent (Malaysia Interview 29, Researcher, REC member) highlights, "[M]y role is not to tell them to be a good Muslim, my role is to tell them how to protect themselves". However, other respondents stated that they were unable to separate their professional obligations from their personal faith obligations, derived from the *Qur'an*, of "enjoining what is right and forbidding what is wrong" (*The Holy Qur'an*, Chapter 3, verse 104). Participants explained how they directly relied on their reading and understanding of the *Qur'an* to guide their decision-making:

> Because, as a Muslim, I think that I have to live in a Islamic framework and consider an Islamic framework for my life. It is very important to see what God says in [the] *Qur'an*. I read every day, trying to find verses of *Holy Qur'an*, and I am trying to consider those verses and those teachings in my life. I think that mostly *Qur'an* is very important in our considerations. To be a Muslim, I am responsible to consider those frameworks for myself, not only in my life, but also in my work and in every aspect of my education and research also.
>
> (Iran Interview 12, Researcher, REC member, guideline developer)

> When you say being ethical, being good, being excellent, it's doing things that [are] according to the teaching of the *Qur'an* and the *Hadith*, in general, for whatever you do. Islam is life. So in research you have to follow the same thing. As long as you follow the teachings of the *Qur'an* and the *Hadith*, that is Islamic.
>
> (Malaysia Interview 1, Researcher, REC member)

The ethical tension that occurs at the personal and professional boundary in relation to the research and health provisions of marginalised groups is two-fold. Participants considered extramarital relations to be outside the legal boundary of Islam, and that they believed they would be morally implicated if they did not address these legal transgressions and, worse still, were associated with the propagation and/or laissez-faire approach to such practices.

Participants, however, described differing views about personal moral and legal culpability, and this has led to tensions. For example, one of the participants in Malaysia described how, in addition to balancing her personal faith and professional obligations, she has faced challenges to her research from colleagues, and she has been questioned for condoning practices considered illicit according to Islamic law:

> I do a wide range of research focusing largely on HIV/AIDS, but also, just a little less, on general infectious disease ... and in HIV/AIDS, I couldn't choose. I mean HIV/AIDS is already controversial, but I couldn't choose to do more non-mainstreaming, in a sense that I do mostly research with the marginalized communities or in the HIV world. It's now called "key affected population". Initially, [we were] mostly focusing on drug users, prisoners. [N] ow, we're also branching into the sex workers and men who have sex with men, so all of the very tabooed, marginalised communities in this country and others ... We come across all the time, with needle exchange and all that, "You're condoning it".
>
> (Malaysia Interview 29, Researcher, REC member)

There is, therefore, a complex interplay between faith and culture in determining moral standards in such contexts. Researchers who decide to undertake work involving marginalised groups need to reconcile many competing personal moral values and also the contextual challenges that are involved in these considerations. She explained that hostilities to her work do not simply come from external organisations and individuals, but also from within the medical profession and from her colleagues. Although she undertook discussions with Islamic scholars who engaged in the process of *ijithad* to derive a *fatwah* that lends approval for her work, she still faces objections from others within the biomedical profession. This points to the fact that there may be limits to the application of *ijtihad* and *fatawah* in addressing such ethical questions.

Participants who personally objected to carrying out and/or approving research on illicit practices explained that they did not consider existing deliberations, offered by the institutional forms of Islam, as sufficient in providing guidance regarding their beliefs about moral culpability. They, thus, clarified that they considered it their religious obligation to oppose such research activities. Again, this points to there being limits to the application of *ijtihad* and *fatawah* in such personal ethical deliberations.

In summary, the above sections indicate that beliefs about intuitions, legal and moral accountability and conscientious objection, which are rooted in religious values, are important when researchers deliberate their role in HIV/AIDS research in such contexts. For some participants, their understanding of their professional obligations to counter epidemics, such as HIV/AIDS, may supersede their personal values and beliefs. Such researchers may take on the role of advocacy for such work, which will now be briefly explored.

Advocacy role of biomedical researchers in the process of ijtihad *and deriving* fatawah *for addressing HIV/AIDS*

It is important to emphasise that, despite the initial challenges in both Malaysia and Iran and the tensions explored above, lobbying from professionals has resulted in engagement from Islamic scholars and the development of ethico-legal analysis that enables research and implementation of needle exchange programmes amongst IVDUs. The data also suggest that it is the biomedical researchers, in such contexts, who have to engage Islamic scholars in order to stimulate health policy shifts. The practical deliberations of researchers and REC members involves them acting as advocates for such work, where these discussions rely on their tabling of such issues. It suggests that such negotiations add an additional layer of complexity to the process of *ijtihad*, as biomedical researchers who participate in this dialectic may take on two roles, that of biomedical experts or contextual scholars with a growing knowledge and commitment to contributing to the Islamic ethico-legal sciences, as well as functioning as advocates for the population they serve and the progress of their profession.

The data suggest that there are particular issues encountered by researchers in Islamic/Muslim contexts who are required to balance two or more moral traditions. These broadly cluster around issues that are either considered illegal within Islamic law or raise theological questions. Tensions occur as these professionals are often trained through a globalised "secular" medical curriculum, and/or they follow or contribute to global biomedical trends and need to reconcile the latter sources of ethical thinking with Islamic ethico-legal elements. Most of the researchers in both countries emphasised that, barring such issues, the ethical questions they face in their work would be shared by researchers globally, and the resources/principles they use are similar to those employed elsewhere.

The analysis shows that Islamic scholars are tasked with the consideration of the overall values and laws that are found within Islam's normative sources to ensure that the process of practical deliberation, through *ijtihad* in producing a *fatwah*, is in harmony with the tradition as well as instructive for practitioners. They have also been given the overall responsibility, authority and title of "scholar", such that it is only after their agreement and endorsement that an edict is considered to have normative value from the perspective of the Islamic legal tradition. The data highlight how Islamic scholars have significant influence over public opinion and what is considered Islamically appropriate. Such influence has been seen to affect health research policy in such contexts. If researchers, therefore, identify a health need that concerns a practice and/or intervention deemed illegal in Islam, scholars would need to be consulted to offer ethico-legal deliberation, through *ijtihad* and a religious endorsement through a *fatwah*, for such interventions to be deemed acceptable.

These different roles and responsibilities of the two groups involved in the process of *ijtihad* leads to tensions, where biomedical researchers explained that there are certain issues that they think are not adequately dealt with by Islamic scholars due to their taboo/illegal nature within the Islamic tradition. Scholars, in turn, explained that they are charged with representing their tradition and need to be mindful of how they employ the legal tradition when undertaking ethico-legal analysis.

Moral consciousness and moral anxiety when researching and meeting the health needs of women

The previous chapter described the ethico-legal challenges that are encountered by researchers who are investigating women's health around domestic and intimate partner violence and women's sexual health and sexual experience. They grapple with national guidelines and professional obligations, through a globalised medical curriculum, that are seemingly gender-neutral,[1] which they negotiate alongside cultural beliefs and values about gender roles, which may be reinforced by "male dominated" scriptural interpretations. The researchers – themselves Muslim – must reconcile these competing interests whilst negotiating their own personal values, which commonly originate from an understanding of their faith. The previous chapters focused on institutional forms of Islam, such as the texts, laws and Islamic scholars, and how they are engaged with and respond to such issues. Here, I will examine in more detail the personal negotiations of respondents, and the practical deliberations they undertake in their direct interaction with participants.

Chapter 5 briefly introduced researchers' moral anxieties, as an emerging theme, when they try to balance the needs and values of their participants alongside their own personal values and professional obligations. An examination of such moral anxieties will be presented here. The data and the experience of one researcher, for example, reveal some deep ethical challenges and questions. As a professional she is keen to meet the standards recommended by guidelines and knows that she ought to respect the views and beliefs of her participants. However, as a Muslim herself, and being familiar with the normative sources and the alternate interpretations regarding the role and status of women in Islam, she is concerned that the women are unable to freely make a decision about whether to enrol in studies investigating intimate and domestic partner violence. The analysis shows that such potential research participants are also anxious and unsure of how much information to disclose, as they are committed to a scriptural interpretation that stipulates that they must keep such issues private.

The researcher is subsequently uncertain of what her professional and personal obligations are. Professionally, she wants to ensure participants are able to freely participate, and she thinks that the freedom to do so would require them to be fully informed of different viewpoints on the role and interpretation of scripture. However, she is aware that such considerations would require a much more

---

1   Chapter 7 will briefly explore the gendered nature of medical knowledge and research. For an excellent account of gendered data bias in medicine and other sciences, please see C. C. Perez. (2019). *Invisible women: Exposing data bias in a world designed for men.* New York: Random House.

extensive investment of time and personnel than are not at her disposal. Yet, she considers the study incredibly important in terms of providing an overview of the extent of the problem of intimate and domestic partner violence in the study populations, their health needs and how the latter can be best addressed through health systems programming. The researcher is also unsure of whether she should simply accept the potential participants' beliefs and values as a mark of respect for there being different interpretations of religious scripture.

She explained how the different obligations she identifies come up against each other, leaving her with a very difficult moral problem of what she ought to do in order to respect, protect and help the victims of abuse:

> [W]hen you talk about obedience, Islam do[es] not want you to just obey without having a real understanding. You do not have to obey your husband who [does not] even practice Islam, for example. Now, how do you tell these women that you're not going against your religion by being disobedient with this person? This disobedience means, basically, for these survivors [who] are really trying to get out or not fulfilling the men's, the perpetrators' desires ... That's why people never talk about rape in a marital relationship, for example. They know it's very painful. It is very hard when you talk to them. They know that, but they just say, "I cannot say no because I'm his wife." How do you impart some knowledge to this person?
>
> I'm very careful when I talk to these survivors, because I've been working with them for a long, long time. How do you tell them in your research that there is a way out from this, so that they can really make a decision, so that they don't have a guilty feeling? That is important for me, that if I engage with the respondent, then the respondent must be confident with that information, and they don't have to have another trauma by feeling guilty, "Oh, I listened to this researcher. Now, I do not know what I have to do, what kind of decision I should make. Should I obey, or should I not obey this?"
>
> You really have to work with that. Of course, that's why researchers, and especially research on women or gender for that matter, always have to have wisdom, because you have to continue working with this respondent so that, whether they agree or disagree with you, they really have a good footing on that decision. It's not just something that they just follow without having real knowledge on that.
>
> (Malaysia Interview 25, Researcher, REC member)

The researcher's experience suggests that she has to negotiate her own deliberations about personal faith and professional obligations as well as consider the tensions participants are balancing in terms of their beliefs and moral conscience about obedience and wanting to participate in the research. She explained how working with such a study population requires ethical considerations beyond safety, confidentiality and privacy. Due to the women's own faith commitments, the researcher explained that she did not want to leave them with feelings of guilt. She suggests that she may need to help research participants come to terms with tensions of personal faith and health needs whilst also negotiating her own deliberations. In the case of the researcher, she considers her professional obligations requiring her to study the prevalence of intimate partner violence whilst ensuring that she is respectful of her participants' beliefs. Her personal faith, however, is driving her to challenge the participants' views. Yet she is concerned that she should only engage in such discussions if she has adequate resources, as she may risk causing more harm to the study participants.

Although she considered that it would be ideal to first educate and "empower" the women, as these changes would require a longer-term intervention, it was difficult to come to an understanding of how to prioritise and plan the research. Should the epidemiological study of enumerating the prevalence of intimate and domestic violence be preceded by some community engagement or education initiative? Or should the former precede the latter, once there is a better understanding of the at-risk group? Further, how should such education be offered, what should the content be, and who should deliver it?

The researcher explained that studying this population meant that the participants needed to have trust in the researcher in order to feel comfortable to discuss "divine concepts" or concepts and values rooted in religious interpretation:

> Practically, when you think of research, for example, you have only that much time doing the research. Women ha[ve] … the respondent must trust you enough to go on further, and you have to develop this trust. For research on values, to engage the respondents on this whole idea of divine concepts and all this, you need to develop that trust to start with. Then, only, you can actually go on and move on into the whole dialogues with them.
>
> (Malaysia Interview 25, Researcher, REC member)

She also explained how, once she embarked on this study, she was unprepared for the follow-up work, as she did not anticipate the support that the women would require, in terms of the anxieties and pain related to their personal relationships with their husbands, or how their beliefs, until they enrolled into the research, may have inadvertently been a coping mechanism. She explained how once they enrolled in the study and began articulating their experiences and concerns, they became more aware of their domestic situation and being accepting of abuse. The researcher explained how she would advise the women in "the intimate partner violence study" that, according to Islamic teachings, obedience to the husband did not extend to the toleration of such abuse. She explained that having started the research and having encountered participants who believed it was their religious duty to obey their husbands and not to disclose the reality of their abuse, she became concerned about the method and implications of her study. She realised the entrenched nature of their beliefs and did not have sufficient funding, personnel or time to set up adequate follow-up and support:

> At that point, basically, I was thinking the weakness … was that we did not set a support network that is strong enough to follow-up with this issue … I

think we didn't expect that as a critical part of the outcome of the research. We did not prepare our colleagues in the NGO to be ready to continue to engage with that debate.

...

What happens is that we acknowledge that this is difficult for the women, the whole context of the values of obedience, for example, because we have one section on values ... Then I realized, as a researcher, you should actually think of the possibilities of setting up the network to support the women for that.

(Malaysia Interview 25, Researcher, REC member)

She then explained further complexities and questions in researching this community, whilst being Muslim herself. The researcher described how, being a committed Muslim, she felt it was her personal obligation to inform victims of abuse that religion cannot be a justification for the violence they had experienced:

Being involved in gender studies, women's rights issues, the first thing that comes to your mind is about empowering these women ... Personally, because I'm a Muslim, I know when, and I deal a lot ... I've been dealing a lot with Muslim survivors themselves. I know they have a lot of issues either with the religious authority [or] with those people in the community. They always find it very difficult express themselves. I see that as part of being believers, in my sisterhood as a Muslim, as practitioners, that I have to share this knowledge with them, not just supporting them because they are in that situation ... I have to share this knowledge ... whatever the Prophet is saying, that, whatever little good thing that you know, you share it with this person. You want to share it so that they can actually see the point, and they can actually build up on that issue. Of course, it's difficult, because you have all men in [the] religious authorities. You're going to be branded as feminist women, or whatever. Whatever. And the women are very scared of you, to some extent, because there is a label about you and your group and your activities and your research.

(Malaysia Interview 25, Researcher, REC member)

She mentioned the Prophetic advice on the virtues and obligations of teaching what one knows of the *Qur'an* (Sahih Bukhari, Book 66, Hadith 49). However, she also explained how, in Malaysia, particularly in the "conservative" states where she works, it is a challenge as a Muslim woman for her to advocate for and research women's health and rights. She explained how such activism may be branded as "feminist" and/or "secular", which may cause the study population to withdraw from such research. She did emphasise that in order for her to carry out the research, it was important for her to engage with the religious authorities on such issues. She described that the challenge she faces with such engagement is that the religious authority mainly consists of men, who do not engage well with such issues. She did, however, state that doing research that is scientifically credible and can be shared with the religious authorities is a first step towards engaging them:

[T]he other thing ... that pushed me into this research is because I want our religious authority to speak with evidence. That was one of the thing that drive[s] me to this research, because I want them to speak with evidence, so that they just don't say, "Oh, no, this is not an issue." I want to give it to them so that they speak with evidence. So, when they engage in a dialogue about these issues in our community, they can actually see the other perspective, the scientific perspective based on research, [and] they can use it. I think this is like another way ... to support the women, by talking to this authority.

(Malaysia Interview 25, Researcher, REC member)

This suggests that her role is not only that of a researcher. As a Muslim woman, she is someone who is also advocating for the participants in her study. A significant challenge she faces doing this work is when she engages with the survivors themselves. She explained how her participants' understanding of "divine concepts" relating to ideas about obedience (*ta'ah*) in the *Qur'an*, as explained in Chapter 5, is influenced by particular interpretations of scripture. When she tries to research the prevalence of domestic and intimate partner violence so she can then bring the data to the attention of religious authorities, victims themselves disagree with enrolment and the nature of the research, as they consider it in conflict with their religious beliefs.

The researcher's concerns and deliberations represent the different roles she is undertaking at one time: researcher, community member, Muslim, educator, advocate and a woman, to name but a few. Is it possible for her to occupy only one or two of these roles at any given time? Can she simply do the research and divorce herself from her personal obligation to provide education and empowerment to women who are victims of abuse? All of these roles are deeply embedded into why she is doing the research, and how she is doing it. Each role also contributes to her moral framework and process of deliberation. Yet, such complex roles and priorities cause her moral anxiety and frustration. The analysis suggests that more research needs to be done to understand the experience of researchers in these contexts and to better understand such moral anxiety.

Conclusions

In summary, the analysis in this chapter indicates, firstly, that the individuals within the institutional forms of Islam, such as biomedical researchers who may act as contextual scholars, are personally struggling with balancing different priorities and value systems, including their own faith. When faced with a practical problem, such as the need to address the HIV/AIDS epidemic or whether and how to enrol women into a research study, the data show that researchers in these contexts concurrently have to consider what is recommended by physicians' codes of conduct, research ethics guidelines, and global health priorities as well as what is instructed by Islam and its formal structures together with local cultural values. The analysis suggests that researchers in such contexts who are required to adopt multiple roles and balance numerous value systems and priorities may face moral anxiety and frustration.

Secondly, in addressing such practical challenges respondents express a deep commitment to Islamic ethics and law, which influences their understanding of their legal and moral accountability. This personal accountability originating from participants' faith commitments adds an additional layer of complexity to the institutional forms of Islam, when the latter are engaged to address the ethical challenges of global health problems like HIV/AIDS. The analysis shows that, despite the institutional forms of Islam legally permitting the use of interventions like needle exchange programmes and condoms for addressing HIV/AIDS, researchers may conscientiously object to employing such interventions due to concerns for their own moral accountability, and/or they may oppose the use of such interventions by others.

Finally, this chapter looks again at the cross-cutting theme of Islamic scholarly authority by analysing the experiences of biomedical researchers and REC members as not only contributors of the contextual information for *ijtihad*, but as drivers or advocates for particular types of research through their professional obligations and understanding of the global biomedical context.

Bibliography

Ahmed, A. & Suleman, M. (2018). Islamic perspectives on the genome and the Human Person: Why the Soul Matters. In M. Ghaly (Ed.). *Islamic ethics and the genome question* (pp. 139–168). Brill.

Ives, J. & Dunn, M. (2010). Who's arguing?: A call for reflexivity in bioethics. *Bioethics*, 24 (5), 256–265.

Rackham, H. (1952). *Aristotle* (Vol. 20). Cambridge, MA: The Loeb Classical Library. Harvard University Press.

Sachedina, A. (2009). *Islamic biomedical ethics: Principles and application*. New York: Oxford University Press.

Sahih Bukhari. Book 66, Hadith 49. http://sunnah.com/bukhari/66/49 (Last accessed 16 June 2016).

Sahih Muslim. Book 22, Hadith 133. https://sunnah.com/muslim/22/133 (Last accessed 5 November 2019).

The Holy Qur'an. Chapter 3, verse 104. http://corpus.quran.com/translation.jsp?chapter=3&verse=104 (Last accessed 28 December 2015).

7 Negotiating multiple moral resources

Key findings and recommendations for future research

The preceding chapters have shown a number of key findings.

Firstly, Islam and its institutional forms do impact ethical decision-making in the day-to-day practice of biomedical research in the countries studied.

Secondly, there are many distinctive mechanisms, such as the involvement of Islamic scholars, the process of *ijtihad* and the production of *fatawah*, by which Islam identifies and develops ethical views about biomedical matters. However, the biomedical issues are sufficiently complex that there are signs that biomedical scientists are increasingly active in using the language and institutional mechanisms of Islam to contribute and help shape these ethical views.

Thirdly, HIV/AIDS poses major challenges to the world of Islam, as it does the rest of world. The ethical issues arising from HIV/AIDS require Islamic responses, as the epidemic raises issues about behavioural practices that are illegal in Islam, such as intravenous drug use, homosexuality and prostitution. This study shows that no simple or single response to the ethical issues arising from HIV/AIDS exists. A range of responses are observed, from the institutional forms of Islam being employed to reinforce or reconfirm values regarding sexual identity through to researchers and scholars finding practical ways to address HIV/AIDS, whilst still respecting Islamic values.

Fourthly, researchers face practical challenges when deliberating women's autonomy in contexts where Islam is appropriated to support certain views and practices. The role and status of women is disputed in such contexts, with views ranging from women needing their husbands' permission to leave the home to men and women having equal freedoms. Researchers also encounter difficulties when researching sensitive issues, such as intimate and domestic partner violence. Challenges to such studies come from many sources, including female participants who are committed to certain scriptural interpretations.

Finally, practical deliberations about ethical issues can often involve tensions between personal and professional values. Researchers, REC members and guideline developers express a deep commitment to Islamic ethics and law, as well as faith-based moral intuitions, which influence their understanding of their legal and moral accountability. When they encounter practical problems, like the ethical issues of HIV/AIDS or women's participation in research, they are tasked with balancing and prioritising different value systems. Muslim researchers may act as advocates for the promotion of needle exchange programmes or contraceptive use based upon the application of the Islamic principle of "public good", or they may conscientiously object to such interventions. Researchers adopt multiple roles and are required to balance numerous value systems and priorities. They face moral anxiety and frustration when these different moral sources are in conflict.

In this chapter I present further reflections on the above findings two through five. The focus is on the tensions, complexities and challenges identified in the data chapters, and I attempt to contextualise these within the broader bioethics and Islamic bioethics literature. The issues and questions raised here will act, I hope, as a primer for future research examining the role of Islam in biomedical research ethics and encouragement for further enquiry into how researchers navigate the complex terrain of international and local guidelines, professional standards, national and global health priorities, cultural influences, institutional forms of Islam as well as their deep, personal understandings of and commitments to faith values. This complex moral nexus remains understudied within bioethics, and as the preceding chapters have shown, the data is incredibly rich and further informs our understanding of how professionals working in contexts where their own religious and cultural commitments, as well as their participants' faith, influence the types of research they undertake and how research is conducted. What the study also shows is that professionals working in such contexts are offered little by way of the current global bioethics discourse that captures their experiences and voices. This lacuna means that we are yet to establish a suitable vocabulary to talk about the types of moral decisions that researchers make in such contexts, the kinds of moral resources they may rely on and how these interact. I hope that this study enriches existing bioethics languages to help us better understand and explain research ethics decision-making in such contexts and enable better training, education and collaboration within and between different settings.

The institutional forms of Islam in biomedical research ethics

Chapter 3 presented an analysis of the array of Islam's institutional aspects in Malaysia and Iran that are involved in the understanding of ethical issues in biomedical research. Concerns relating to Islam are raised at multiple levels and addressed differently in each of the countries I visited: more centrally in Iran, due to the political establishment of an Islamic state, and through a parallel system in Malaysia, via state-level *Shariah* courts, national/state-level *fatwah* councils and/ or individually consulted Islamic scholars (*muftis*). The elements of Islam and its normative sources that influence ethical thinking within biomedical research include, but are not limited to, the foundational texts (*Qur'an* and *Hadith*), the *Shariah* (Islamic law), *fiqh* (Islamic jurisprudence), *ijtihad* (independent reasoning) to arrive at *fatawah* (legal edicts) and the involvement of Islamic scholars. When issues that are considered relevant to Islamic law and theology emerge, in both countries Islamic scholars are consulted to review whether there is instruction within the normative sources of Islam (*Qur'an, Hadith, Shariah*, legal precedent in courts, *fatawah*) to direct what ought to be done. If there is no answer in the normative sources, then the scholars are required to undertake independent reasoning, or *ijtihad*, which is a process that incorporates two components to enable them to arrive at a *fatwah*. The first component for *ijtihad* is the contextual information about what the ethico-legal issue is, how it has arisen and what its implications may be. The second component is the review of the overall values and instructions that Islamic scholars glean from Islam's normative sources to ensure that they arrive at an ethico-legal instruction (*fatwah*) about what ought to be done in light of Islam's normative sources.

This study has shown that scholarly engagement and the employment of *ijtihad* are used for issues that pose theological and/or legal concerns in Islam. Such issues may require national consultation, for example, for the authorisation of stem cell research, while others are raised as individual concerns, such as researchers consulting scholars for the approval of a porcine-based vaccine for a study. The adaptability of Islam's institutional elements in the consideration of ethical issues in research, as indicated by the case study, shows that the overall system is flexible and works to meet the demands of those within it in a pragmatic and innovative fashion. However, there are constraints. Although the involvement of Islamic scholars and the instruction derived from Islam's normative sources has been largely flexible and permissive, there are limitations and complexities that emerge around the issue of Islamic scholarly authority.

Although the task of *ijtihad* and issuing *fatawah* has been seen traditionally as the role of Islamic scholars, one of the striking features of the data analysis in this study is that there is increasing involvement from biomedical experts (contextual scholars who are also informally trained in the Islamic sciences) and "bridge-scholars" (those formally trained in biomedicine and the Islamic sciences) in this practical reasoning process in the context of biomedical research. These emerging scholars provide the contextual information for *ijtihad*. They have also been equipping themselves with the language and knowledge of the Islamic sciences to contribute to the second component – consideration of what the Islamic normative sources would instruct. This study shows that, although the formal label and recognition of Islamic scholarly authority is still reserved for those trained formally in the Islamic sciences, the debate about ethical issues is increasingly involving the input of biomedical experts and "bridge scholars". There are, however, tensions and challenges arising from this evolution of Islamic scholarly authority and deliberation.

Some of the challenges include traditional scholars being unfamiliar with the contextual complexities of research and biomedical advancement. The data have shown that in both countries, traditional scholars are called upon to provide religious rulings either through legal or political requirement or personal need. So, within the field of biomedical research ethics, this study has shown that Islamic scholars are keen to work in collaboration with biomedical experts to arrive at an informed ethico-legal decision. This method is in keeping with what has been described in the Islamic bioethics literature, where scholars of the text and context deliberate over emerging bioethical problems (Ramadan, 2009, pp. 1–50; Ghaly, 2013a; Padela, 2007; Shabana, 2014).

Studies have shown that Muslim medical and scientific experts are keen to adopt the language of Islamic theology and law (Ghaly, 2013a) to draft Islamic legal rulings in an attempt to answer emerging religio-ethical challenges. Ghaly, (2013a) suggests that the role of biomedical experts in the process of *ijtihad* is not limited to presenting scientific information. They also contribute by presenting "the human rights discourse pertinent to people living with HIV/AIDS, [giving] an account of the preventive strategy adopted by the WHO, and offer[ing] an [Islamic] virtue-based preventive model" (Ghaly, 2013a, p. 617). Such contributions by biomedical experts were also observed in both case study sites. However, this study shows that, beyond being concerned for technical accuracy within the process of *ijtihad* and offering human-rights-based or virtue-based models of care, biomedical experts are keen to get more involved, as there are concerns about information sharing and transparency in the production of *fatawah*.

Many of the participants were very well versed in the Islamic foundational texts and sciences. They were keen to not only present their contextual knowledge within such consultations, but also their understanding and opinion of the normative texts and what the subsequent rulings ought to be. The keenness of biomedical experts to adopt this normative role has been described in collaborations involving other Islamic bioethical issues, such as beginning of life (Ghaly, 2015). This study shows that biomedical experts within the context of research are taking on a similar role. It is evident from this study that the expanding function of biomedical experts in contributing to both elements of *ijtihad* has led to tensions regarding the authority of issuing *fatawah*. In both Malaysia and Iran there is consensus that only Islamic scholars hold this authority. The data within this study has shown that such a view of Islamic authority is leading to tensions within collaborations. Biomedical experts feel there is a lack of transparency about how scholars arrive at their rulings and whether scholars should be afforded such authority when they rely so heavily on the expertise and knowledge of others.

The latter concern has also been described in the literature. Ghaly (2015) suggests a co-mufti role for contextual experts, such as biomedical researchers, where the process of *ijtihad* is considered collective, and the role of contextual experts is not simply consultative. Such an arrangement may theoretically place the three types of scholars (Islamic, contextual and bridge scholars) on the same level when they have to work together, in practice, to resolve the dilemmas they encounter. However, it is unclear how such a shift in the recognition and authority of contextual and bridge scholars would be implemented, or what the impact of such a shift would be. Consideration of these issues is beyond the scope of this study, but they may be addressed by future research.

Overall, however, conferring of a shared authority to contextual and bridge scholars may be a possible means of addressing some of the concerns emerging from this research around information sharing and transparency in the process of *ijtihad*. Contextual and bridge scholars may also feel their contributions are better valued, and this may alleviate some of the tensions seen in the interactions between the three types of scholars. Cooperation and transparency in the collaboration between these experts may ensure that the subsequent *fatawah* are relevant. It may offer more clarity for biomedical researchers, REC members and guideline developers who are seeking guidance about what they should do in the context of specific ethical problems. Such a process may also strengthen the normative weight of Islamic scholarly authority and *fatawah* where biomedical researchers, who are keen to act harmoniously with their faith, are able to better understand and access deliberations that are informed both by textual and contextual knowledge. The mechanism may also play a role in alleviating some of the individual, personal moral tensions and anxieties that researchers encounter when negotiating different moral resources that do not concur. Yet, whether such a collaboration and shared authority is feasible in the context of biomedical research, and what the impact of such an arrangement would be will require further study.

Islamic responses to the ethical issues of HIV/AIDS

Chapter 4 described and analysed how the ethical issues arising from HIV/AIDS require Islamic responses, as the epidemic raises issues about behavioural practices that are illegal in Islam. Commitments to the *Shariah* and its underlying normative sources, the *Qur'an* and *Hadith*, are evident from the data. In both countries, what is clearly outlined as illegal in the source texts is not contested. Matters considered illicit within the *Shariah* encountered in the study include the use of harmful substances, such as IV drugs; alcohol use; extramarital sex and homosexuality. Although it is contested by some whether the latter issues are illegal, there is general consensus amongst legal experts and lay people what Islamic law indicates in relation to these issues (Ghaly, 2013a). Padela (2007) explains that, within the broader Islamic bioethics literature, ethico-legal analysis is closely tied to the boundaries of the *Shariah*.

The institutional forms of Islam are formally engaged with in order to address the ethical issues of HIV/AIDS. In particular, Islamic scholars are trying to address the ethical issues through the process of *ijtihad* to derive *fatawah*. This research shows that *ijtihad* and the development of *fatawah* have been key in stimulating or endorsing a re-evaluation of the ethical issues of HIV/AIDS, which are perceived in a negative light due to their being illegal in Islam. This study highlights that the process of *ijtihad* and production of *fatawah* are distinct and recognisably important means of ethico-legal deliberation in Islamic contexts. Although, initially, there was resistance to accepting the health needs of IVDUs in both countries, there was engagement from Islamic scholars and subsequent agreement that researching and implementing needle exchange programmes ought to be accepted. This study offers a more substantive account of the ethical issues emerging from HIV/AIDS research, including how "public good" is understood through the process of *ijtihad* to derive *fatawah* in Malaysia and Iran in order to instruct researchers on what ought to be done in the case of IVDUs and needle exchange programmes. It suggests that the Islamic-ethico-legal system is flexible and permissive enough to deal with the tensions that arise as a result of pressures of global health and global health policy. It also presents this mechanism as being distinct in the two countries due to their theological-philosophical traditions. Other studies have discussed similar engagement of Islamic scholars in the deliberations around IVDUs and needle exchange programmes; however, their focus has been health policy and practice, rather than research (Kamarulzaman & Saifuddeen, 2010; Ghaly, 2013a).

The study also illustrates that, despite the permissive and flexible mechanism of practical deliberation offered by *ijtihad* in producing *fatawah*, tensions exist in the consideration of the health needs of sex workers and the LGBT community in Malaysia and Iran. The findings are in keeping with other studies conducted, not on HIV/AIDS research, but on health policy and practice. They suggest that Islam "plays an important role in shaping health policies and strategies related to HIV prevention in Malaysia" (Barmania & Aljunid, 2016, p. 1), and there are differences of opinion amongst biomedical researchers and Islamic scholars about how the ethical issues of HIV/AIDS ought to be addressed. What this study adds is that there is provision within Islamic law to enable deliberations about these ethical issues and to grant permissions for condom use, including the principles of "public good" (*maslaha*) and "preservation of life" (one of the *maqasid* or objectives of the *Shariah*). However, there has been concern from Islamic scholars and biomedical experts alike that abstinence is the recognised Islamic way of curtailing spread of disease and research on the use of condoms signifies acceptance of illicit practices. Continuing efforts from Islamic scholars, biomedical experts and bridge-scholars deliberating such global health challenges may stimulate a re-evaluation of these issues. This gap may also point to there being a limit to the application of the process of *ijtihad* and the development of *fatawah* as a tool of ethico-legal deliberation for such issues. More research needs to be done to understand the socio-cultural challenges underlying barriers to condom use amongst sex workers and MSMs as well as to monitor the levels of engagement of the three types of scholars who are deliberating such issues in these contexts.

Women's participation in biomedical research

I investigated how the question of women's autonomy is an ethical problem for researchers in such contexts and how Islam's institutional forms are appropriated to support and/or maintain certain views and practices in relation to the roles and status of women. Disagreements can also be found in the literature, where some authors suggest that "the woman in Islam represents the cornerstone of the family, and it is the responsibility of a man to ensure her protection and welfare" (Afifi, 2007, p. 382). The application of this protection is seen in the requirement that researchers seek "the approval of the family" (Afifi, 2007, p. 382) before enrolling a Muslim female participant. Others, however, argue that "patriarchal" interpretations of the *Qur'an* and *Hadith* have led to such views and, in fact, Islam emphasizes fairness between women and men (Ramadan, 2009, pp. 207–32). Some participants in this study, including Islamic scholars, also shared the latter view. In both countries, at the level of researchers and RECs, the data show that there is a variation in understanding of what ought to be done when enrolling women in research and the types of studies involving women's health that can be undertaken.

What also emerged from the data is that the notion of autonomy understood by some researchers in Malaysia and Iran is different to that understood in the "Western" secular construct. The data analysis suggests that the Islamic tradition does not focus on the individual, but on their relationship with God. Decision-making also is not focused on the individual, but the family. This is in line with other studies that have called for a reassessment of the understanding and application of the principle of autonomy in Islamic contexts (Afifi, 2007). However, this study shows that such understandings of autonomy come up against notions of *Wilayah* (guardianship), *Qiwammah* (authority), *Ta'ah* (obedience) and *Nushuz* (disobedience). The analysis shows that differing interpretations of the latter terms raise ethical tensions and challenges for researchers, particularly when investigating domestic and intimate partner violence or the sexual health and sexual experience of women.

Chapter 1 highlighted that some authors, such as Macklin, have expressed concerns about extreme versions of moral relativism undermining values that are universal, such as human rights (Macklin, 1999, p. 24), and the understanding and application of principles like autonomy. In this study the data suggests that, although religion and culture play a significant role in determining people's individual and collective moral universes, when religion is appropriated to lend authority to "male-dominated" or patriarchal structures, values and beliefs, it may lead to ethical challenges for researchers and RECs. Macklin's apprehensions about the overreach of, for example, religion and/or culture in determining moral deliberations in such contexts becomes particularly relevant (Macklin, 1999, p. 24) as the women who are affected by the religious legitimisation of cultural patriarchy are rarely able to challenge status quo. Nor is it clear in such contexts who represents their interests, if at all. Furthermore, as the women themselves are deeply faithful, they not only adhere to but also protect or advocate for a patriarchal order, as they are convinced the norms are rooted in religion. The study findings likewise reveal that religious beliefs are also crucial for victims as coping mechanisms. When they are challenged about their views, victims experience distress and isolation.

Although we may consider researchers encountering such values and belief systems as being faced with the difficult challenge of practically negotiating universal and relative norms, this study shows that a polychotomy, not a dichotomy, is at play. Researchers' experiences reveal that their empirical reality is more complex. Their deliberations do not involve alternative moral sources, they involve multiple moral sources. In such contexts, analysing the ethical reality of researchers through binary tropes like universalism or relativism may prevent us from appreciating fully the deep and complex moral universe within which they reside. The study also shows that there is an opportunity to expand our current bioethics vocabulary by embracing the moral lens through which researchers in such contexts deliberate. Pluralising our resources and what is meant by "good research" in such contexts may better enable us to disentangle the underlying complexity of women's autonomy and ensure their safety and appropriate enrolment and engagement in research.

For example, this study underlines that there are particular verses of the *Qur'an* and passages of *Hadith* that are called on more frequently for supporting views that favour male "guardianship" and "authority". Islamic scholars have called for a re-evaluation of such interpretations of scripture (Ramadan, 2009, pp. 207–32). Participants' concerns about the role of the family emphasizes, however, that such reinterpretations may need to offer sufficient respect to the normative texts of Islam and their overall emphasis on the family over the individual (Ramadan, 2009, pp. 207–32). Although some of these contested references in the *Qur'an* and *Hadith* are highlighted in this study, more research is required in this area.

A recent re-examination of such *Quranic* verses from a woman's perspective, whilst referring to the pre-existing tradition (Wadud, 1999, pp. 74–5), explains that the terms *nushuz* cannot mean "disobedience to the husband", as it refers to both the man and the woman; it is more likely to refer to "marital disharmony". Also Wadud's seminal work suggests that "*daraba*" does not mean "to hit", as has been commonly understood; rather, it can mean, as suggested by some of the scholars I interviewed, "to set as an example" or "to leave" (Wadud, 1999, p. 76). Overall, Wadud suggests that the *Qur'an* is pointing to methods of dealing with marital disharmony rather than pointing individually to the man or woman and, more importantly, suggesting or condoning violence against women. The latter would be against the overall spirit of the *Qur'an* and, there-fore, would contradict accepted methods of *Quranic* interpretation. Wadud explains that the problem of domestic violence in Muslim families is "not rooted in this *Quranic* passage" (Wadud, 1999, p. 76). She explains that the men who hit their wives are not seeking marital harmony, rather they are simply motivated to harm (Wadud, 1999, p. 76). Such scholarship is transforming the Islamic tradition, and it is challenging the notion of Islam justifying such violence. Wadud's work and that of other scholars, such as Khaled Aboul Fadl (El Fadl, 2014), suggest that the normative sources of Islam have been appropriated to reinforce cultural views and practices. This study suggests that more work needs to be done to explore the impact of this complex interaction of religion and culture in the context of biomedical research ethics. Some of the themes pre-sented may help to add layers of complexity to existing discussions around uni-versalism and relativism within the bioethics discourse.

Practical deliberations involving personal and professional values

This study has shown that the individuals within the institutional forms of Islam, such as biomedical researchers who may act as contextual scholars, are personally struggling with balancing different priorities and value systems, including their own faith. When faced with a practical problem, such as the need to address the HIV/AIDS epidemic or whether and how to enrol women into a research study, the data show that researchers in these contexts concurrently have to consider what is recommended by physicians' codes of conduct, research ethics guidelines, global health priorities, as well as what is instructed by Islam and its formal struc-tures together with local cultural values. This study suggests that researchers in such contexts, who are required to adopt multiple roles and balance numerous value systems and priorities, may face moral anxiety and frustration.

Also, in addressing such practical challenges, respondents express a deep commitment to Islamic ethics and law, which influences their understanding of their legal and moral accountability. Personal accountability, which originates from participants' faith commitments, adds an additional layer of complexity to the institutional forms of Islam when the latter are engaged to address the ethical challenges of global health problems like HIV/AIDS. The data show that, despite the institutional forms of Islam legally permitting the research and use of interventions like needle exchange programmes and condoms for addressing HIV/AIDS, researchers may conscientiously object to researching and employing such interventions due to concerns for their own moral accountability, and/or they may oppose the use of such interventions by others.

Deliberations by biomedical experts in such contexts also point to them being not only contributors of the contextual information for *ijtihad*, but also drivers or advocates for particular types of research through their professional obligations and understanding of the global biomedical context. The data also suggest that, while some biomedical researchers may act as advocates for such health interventions, others, due to their own understanding of Islamic law and personal faith, reject and directly oppose the implementation of such interventions.

The study suggests that the participants' understanding of Islam is not a predictable, monochrome, linear script of moral deliberation; rather, it comprises of a rich set of sources, values and virtues that constantly have to be interpreted and negotiated based on contextual and textual (Islamic scriptural) realities at any given time. The Islamic sources, their interpretation and application do not produce a predictable read out or a script of what the ethical answer is to any problem. It has to be constantly negotiated within its religio-cultural context at the personal level.

This study points, therefore, to broader implications for bioethics. In practice, researchers are not able to simply consider and enact a bioethical principle or Islamic ethico-legal guidance. Rather, what they do is have these principles running alongside other values, preferences and competing influences that enable them to arrive at a personal ethical decision in any given context. This personal deliberation also involves an important process of consultation with others, such as colleagues and experts. It points to a type of moral particularism being evident in Islamic contexts, which requires further study. Blum explains that, within the existing bioethics literature, there is very little consideration given to moral perception and particularity (Blum, 1994, pp. 30–44). Although much is said about guidelines and rules, there is little deliberation about how a situation may "have a particular character for a particular moral agent" (Blum, 1994, p. 30). Dancy explains that ethical narratives may not be narrowed into "a principle" per se, and what is considered a reason to act in one situation need not be considered the reason in another case (Dancy, 2004, pp. 1–12). Few studies within the broader bioethics discourse have been carried out to analyse "the who" of bioethics – "who are the individuals tasked with bioethics", and who are at "frontline of face-to-face interactions with medical research participants" (Kingori, 2013, p. 361).

No studies have been done to date to explore the moral universe of the Muslim researcher and/or researchers who work within Islamic/Muslim contexts. Looking at the moral world of respondents, by exploring the influence of Islam as a personal faith, has been a way to better understand how Islam influences ethical decision-making of researchers, REC members, guideline developers and Islamic scholars in the biomedical research context. Against that background, this empirical study is a first attempt at capturing the complexity encountered by researchers in Islamic contexts and the dilemmas that arise when personal motivations and values come up against those required by professional commitments. More research needs to be done to understand this interaction better.

It is important to briefly mention here that such tensions are not limited to the Islamic faith. People of other faith traditions, who are required to reconcile personal moral views, moral guidelines and professional guidelines, also encounter such challenges. One such example is within Christianity, as discussed in Catholic bioethics. Scholars such as Engelhardt (2000, pp. 129–34) and Duffy (1988) describe the moral challenges of devising and implementing "non-discriminatory policies" in relation to HIV/AIDS, where healthcare professionals may have to "rethink the meaning of sexual responsibility" (Duffy, 1988, p. 190). Numerous studies in sub-Saharan Africa, including Nigeria (Smith, 2004) and Kenya (Forsyth et al., 1996), describe the difficulties researchers and healthcare professionals face in trying to reconcile multiple moral sources. Future work may be able to further elaborate on these shared challenges and analyse what could be learned about the moral deliberations and compromises from people of different faith traditions.

Summary of key contributions of this study and future research

This study aimed to explore how Islam influences ethical decision-making of researchers, REC members, guideline developers and Islamic scholars in the biomedical research context. As there have been no empirical studies carried out in Malaysia or Iran to investigate the types of issues that emerge when Islam and its normative elements influence biomedical research ethics, this work may be important for local researchers, REC members and guideline developers because it draws attention to a range of issues, which have been captured in the study, and some reasons why such issues may arise in their given context.

Many of the elements included within the methods and analysis of this research are understudied, including biomedical research ethics in Malaysia and Iran, the role and status of women in Islam and within health research, research involving marginalised groups in Islamic contexts and the identification of how the broader Islamic ethico-legal system, its values and edicts arise and impact the understanding of ethics in research. The study also includes a guideline review, which incorporates the analysis of documents and resources that have not previously been studied. This study is, to my knowledge, the first of its kind. It provides stakeholder perspectives – researchers, REC members, guideline developers, bridge scholars and Islamic scholars – to better understand the complexity of views and challenges in relation to Islam and biomedical research ethics.

Despite the contextual limitations, in terms of what can be generalised from this study, the broader analysis of the ethico-legal issues arising from HIV/AIDS, sexuality and sexual health research; women's participation in research; and authority in Islam and its influence on biomedical research potentially has implications for the wider Islamic bioethical discourse. The empirical study highlights that, in these two contexts, ethical issues arising from concerns about authority in Islam, intricacies and conflicts between religion and culture and the appropriation of Islam to authorise certain views, which challenges the ability of health professionals to research, advocate and address the health needs of marginalised groups, point to the need for further investigation in other settings.

This study also highlights possible approaches and emerging questions for further researching ethico-legal concerns arising from the above topics, including consideration of the role of co-muftiship of contextual scholars within biomedical research ethics, training and involvement of bridge scholars, elucidation of a better understanding of the legal boundary of Islam and whether and how Islam should impact the understanding of ethics in biomedical research. The study also suggests a need to further research the complex interaction between culture and religion in the context of biomedical research ethics. Such issues and approaches may need to be better incorporated and studied within the broader fields of Islamic ethics and bioethics.

The qualitative methodology employed was ideal for capturing and further exploring issues involving Islam that participants offered as being morally problematic within their work. The study shows that most participants are able to address the day-to-day moral questions arising from their work in a pragmatic way, which combines their different moral resources to balance personal values and faith commitments alongside professional obligations to their research participants and the wider biomedical field/community. In terms of the broader field of bioethics, normative work to evaluate whether such contexts may benefit from incorporating religio-ethical training within the standard bioethical training may be considered. Also, the normative question arising from this study, whether culture ought to be identified as distinct from religion when the latter is appropriated to authorise the former, may build on existing universalism versus relativism discussions within bioethics. Similarly, by illustrating the complexity and personalised nature of ethical decision-making in such contexts, this study provides empirical insights into moral particularism and points to the need for further research to better understand the formulation of particularism within the Islamic context.

Finally, this study has provided a rich sociological account about the ways in which debates and questions involving Islam within the biomedical research context are negotiated and solved, as well as where some of the gaps are in the thinking and practice of bioethics in such contexts. This is currently lacking within the broader bioethics literature, in terms of our understanding of the Islamic perspective in deliberating, articulating and addressing such issues. It also sets up the question of what needs to be done from the lessons and challenges outlined by the participants interviewed in the study and through my own analysis of the Islamic ethico-legal discourse. What also must be emphasised here is that, although the topics chosen within this study were a prism through which the ethico-legal issues arising from the influence of Islam on biomedical research were explored, these topics and related questions and concerns are not internal to Islam. The marginalisation of women and the prejudice and abuse faced by groups, such as sex workers and those from the LGBT community, are relevant not only for biomedical research ethics, but also for broader discussions within global health and human rights. This suggests that the empirical findings of this study are applicable in other areas, and they can be used to inform other studies seeking to investigate and address some of these ethical challenges.

Although there are many limitations to this study, some of which that are highlighted in Chapter 8, it is hoped that this piece of work will inform the future of this nascent field. I also trust that the richer understanding of the contexts provided by this study will serve as an evidence base for more philosophical and theological thinking on issues in research ethics in Islamic contexts.

Bibliography

Afifi, R. Y. (2007). Biomedical research ethics: An Islamic view. Part II. *International Journal of Surgery*, 5(6), 381–383.

Barmania, S. & Aljunid, S. M. (2016). Navigating HIV prevention policy and Islam in Malaysia: Contention, compatibility or reconciliation? Findings from in-depth interviews among key stakeholders. *BMC Public Health*, 16(1), 524.

Blum, L. A. (1994). *Moral perception and particularity.* Cambridge: Cambridge University Press.

Dancy, J. (2004). *Ethics without principles.* Cambridge: Oxford University Press on Demand.

Duffy, M. F. (1988). The challenge to the Christian community. *Religious Education*, 83 (2), 190–199.

El Fadl, K. A. (2014). *Speaking in God's name: Islamic law, authority and women.* Oxford: Oneworld Publications.

Engelhardt, H. T. (2000). *The foundations of Christian bioethics.* Lisse, The Netherlands: Swets & Zeitlinger.

Forsythe, S., Rau, B., Alrutz, N., Gold, E., Hayman, J. & Lux, L. (1996). *AIDS in Kenya: Socioeconomic impact and policy implications.* http://www.popline.org/node/301833 (Last accessed 7 May 2017).

Ghaly, M. (2013a). Collective religio-scientific discussions on Islam and HIV/AIDS: I. Biomedical scientists. *Zygon®*, 48(3), 671–708.

Ghaly, M. (2015). Biomedical scientists as co-muftis: Their contribution to contemporary Islamic bioethics. *Die Welt des Islams*, 55(3–4), 286–311.

Kamarulzaman, A. & Saifuddeen, S. M. (2010). Islam and harm reduction. *International Journal of Drug Policy*, 21(2), 115–118.

Kingori, P. (2013). Experiencing everyday ethics in context: Frontline data collectors perspectives and practices of bioethics. *Social Science & Medicine*, 98, 361–370. doi:10.1016/j.socscimed.2013.10.013.

Macklin, R. (1999). *Against relativism: Cultural diversity and the search for ethical universals in medicine.* New York: Oxford University Press.

Padela, A. I. (2007). Islamic medical ethics: A primer. *Bioethics*, 21(3), 169–178.

Ramadan, T. (2009). *Radical reform: Islamic ethics and liberation*. New York: Oxford University Press.

Shabana, A. (2014). Bioethics in Islamic thought. *Religion Compass*, 8(11), 337–346.

Smith, D. J. (2004). Youth, sin and sex in Nigeria: Christianity and HIV/AIDS-related beliefs and behaviour among rural-urban migrants. *Culture, Health & Sexuality*, 6(5), 425–437.

Wadud, A. (1999). *Qur'an and woman: Re-reading the sacred text from a woman's perspective* (2nd ed.). New York: Oxford University Press.

8 Methodological annexe

This chapter provides a detailed account of the methods employed during the research. It outlines the rationale of the chosen research sites, followed by an account of the types of data that were needed to conduct an empirical study and the qualitative research method that was employed to gather and analyse the data. The empirical study involved data collection via the qualitative method of semi-structured interviews and a framework analysis. In addition to the data analysis, an ethical analysis was also carried out, the rationale and method for which will be presented here. I have also attempted to include the shortcomings of each of the methodological steps, including the guideline review. I hope that inclusion of this detailed methodology will act as a resource for junior researchers seeking to undertake similar research in the liminal space between bioethics and social science.

Rationale for chosen research sites

The sampling of possible research sites was limited to the OIC in order to maximise the opportunity to evaluate the influence of Islam on the decision-making of biomedical researchers. It was considered more suitable to carry out the study in countries that formally identify themselves as being members of the "Muslim world".[1] Additionally, I was keen to carry out the empirical study in countries that were found to have research ethics guidelines (see Chapter 2) and were, therefore, likely to have research ethics infrastructures, such as ethics committees. The guideline review revealed that, of the 57 OIC countries, only 21 have laws and guidelines relating to research ethics and structures relevant to research ethics (18 available in English).

I systematically contacted the 21 ministries of health of these countries to request their relevant guidelines and codes and permission to conduct in-depth interviews at their research institutions. The countries of focus were those with a significant Muslim population, and those that would be agreeable to a DPhil

---

1 Organisation of Islamic Cooperation. (2015). Organisation of Islamic Cooperation: The collective voice of the Muslim world. http://www.oic-oci.org/page/?p_id= 52&p_ref=26&lan=en (Last accessed 25 October 2015).

candidate conducting a study of their approach to research ethics. After an initial email was sent to the ministries, I sent a follow-up email after a month if I had not received a reply. Most (14) did not reply. I received kind emails from Saudi Arabia, Indonesia and Bangladesh, however, each of the ministries said that they could not support my research. I received positive responses from Iran, Malaysia and Uganda. Although ethics approval was successfully sought from all three countries, given the constraints of time and resources, the study was limited to fieldwork in Iran and Malaysia. Although Uganda also would have been a valuable site for study, it has a minority Muslim population. Because both Iran and Malaysia have significant Muslim populations, it was deemed more suitable to conduct the empirical work there. It was considered more likely that the influence of Islam on biomedical research ethics would be appreciable in a country where Islam is the predominant faith and they have formally declared themselves as "Islamic" through their membership in the OIC.

Iran and Malaysia, therefore, met all of the following country-selection criteria:

- A Muslim majority
- Involvement in biomedical research
- Presence of research ethics guidelines and ethics committees
- Amenable to a DPhil candidate conducting a study on the influence of Islam on biomedical research ethics.

Through local contacts in Malaysia and Iran, suitable permissions were obtained, and the means for participant recruitment and the infrastructure for data collection through interviews were organised. The identification of case study sites, therefore, mixed pragmatism and rational choices, based on which countries provided the necessary permissions, a Muslim majority and a research ethics infrastructure.

I will now briefly outline the historical and contemporary religio-political contexts of Malaysia and Iran. The two sites offer contrasting organisations of Islamic authority and complex histories of personal religiosity and state-level Islamisation, making them ideal sites for this study.

Malaysia: A brief historical and contemporary overview of the socioeconomic and religio-ethnic context

Malaysia, a country in South East Asia (SEA) with a population of 30 million (Hock, 2007, p 165), is striving to achieve developed nation status by 2020 (Tan et al., 2010). Benefitting from political stability following independence from British colonial rule, Malaysia has become a key economic player in SEA (Drabble & Booth, 2000, pp. 1–50) and amongst the OIC countries. With a burgeoning economy, Malaysia has been keen to conduct clinical research and serve as a site for outsourced clinical trials. It has become a popular site for industry and government sponsored trials because the trial process has been found to be cheaper, with faster recruitment of participants (Gross & Hirose, 2007; Glickman et al.,

2009). However, some authors have suggested that one of the reasons for the outsourcing of clinical trials to countries like Malaysia is to avoid the rigorous governance mechanisms present in source countries (Yusuf, 2014; Garrafa et al., 2010). With growing interest and suitable infrastructure for conducting research in neighbouring countries, such as Thailand and Singapore (Korieth & Anderson, 2013), Malaysia has recently had to rethink its health research infrastructure to ensure a favourable system for foreign sponsored trials. The following is a brief overview of the historical and contemporary role of Islam in Malaysia, and why the country was deemed a suitable site for this study.

The arrival of Islam in the Malay Archipelago

The expansion of Islam during the 13th and 15th centuries (Hodgson, 1977b, pp. 543–51) saw its spread to the southern seas and the Malay straits. Sea trade in the region led to the settlement of Muslim sailors and merchants. In the late 13th century, the first Islamic sultanate was established in the Sumatran side of the straits (Hodgson, 1977b, pp. 543–51). However, Islam became politically established within the Malay straits in the 13th century during the Malacca sultanate of Megat Iskandar Shah (ruled from 1414–1424), the second Sultan of Malacca, when he became the first Malay ruler to convert to Islam (Hooker & Osborne, 2003, pp. 58–77). Malacca, on the Malay peninsula side of the straits, was then the strongest port in the region (Hodgson, 1977b, pp. 543–51). Iskander Shah's attraction to the Islamic faith is explained by the widespread acceptance of the Persianised rulership of the Abbasid dynasty (8th to 13th centuries), with the establishment of Muslim sultanates across the Middle East and the Indian Subcontinent by the 15th century (Hooker & Osborne, 2003, pp. 58–77). Traders from these sultanates travelled to SEA, passing through the Straits of Malacca and bringing with them their practices of Islam. The Malay Archipelago has been described as being receptive during this time to the predominant political culture of medieval Islam (Hooker & Osborne, 2003, pp. 58–77). During the Abbasid dynasty, the solidarity afforded to traders by the growing Muslim empire attracted merchants to Islam, and its political expression won the favour of the rulers (Hooker & Osborne, 2003, pp. 58–77). Iskander Shah's establishment of Islam as the state religion became widely known in the rest of the Muslim world, and Malacca became renowned as a trade centre that upheld Muslim values, respected Muslim law and protected fellow Muslims (Hooker & Osborne, 2003, pp. 58–77). Soon after the Malay straits accepted Islam, the surrounding archipelago followed (Hodgson, 1977b, pp. 543–51).

The changing role of Islamic law and the Shariah courts in the peri-colonial period

From the 15th century to the peri-colonial period, the law applied in Malaysia was Islamic law or *Shariah*, accompanied by elements of native Malay custom (Kamali, 1997). There are, however, few primary sources to inform us of the legal and political systems of this period (Shuaib, 2012). Rare surviving documentation, according to researchers, lists forms of Islamic law that were applied in the region within the pre-colonial period (Shuaib, 2012). During the colonial era, however, the legal system that was established followed a more pluralistic model of federal law based on English law (Shuaib, 2012), thus altering the influence and application of *Shariah* in the region. The application of the *Shariah* was further challenged during the colonial era to ensure that "the Islamic law was not interpreted and applied in a manner that conflicted with British understandings of justice, [and] residents tried to ensure that decisions from Islamic courts could be appealed to civil courts staffed by British trained judges" (Shuaib, 2012, p. 89).

When the state of Malaysia was created in 1957, the constitution established a federal system where the majority of judicial power resided within the federal courts, and few aspects of Muslim life were governed within the *Shariah* courts under Islamic law. Following independence, Malaysia comprises 14 states, 12 in West Malaysia and 2 in East Malaysia. Nine of the 14 states are governed by a sultan, and these are assigned largely according to a hereditary monarchy. Politically, the ruling party and prime minister govern the country and hold executive power. The king is the head of state and signs off on legislation but does not hold executive power.[2] The religious structure in Malaysia is organised both at the federal and state level. At the federal level, the king is head, and the National *Fatwah* Council holds executive power. At the state level, the sultan is head, and the state *Mufti* holds executive power. States with no hereditary sultan take the king as their religious head (Shuaib, 2012). A schematic diagram of the political and religious structures in Malaysia is presented in Figure 8.1.

Islamic revival in Malaysia

When Malaysia was founded, each of the states was given the constitutional right[3] to be able to identify and adjudicate matters relating to Muslim citizens within the *Shariah* courts according to Islamic law. However, the subordination of the *Shariah* courts to the civil courts meant that the former were only able to regulate a limited range of domestic and personal concerns recorded

2   Constitution of Malaysia. Part IV – The Federation, Chapter 3 – The executive. http://www1.umn.edu/humanrts/research/malaysia-constitution.pdf (Last accessed 15 January 2020).
3   Constitution of Malaysia (1957). Ninth schedule, Legislative lists, List II – State list. http://www.commonlii.org/my/legis/const/1957/24.html (Last accessed 15 January 2020).

Political Structure

National level
    Head of state   Executive Power
      King   *Parliament and prime minister*

....

Religious structure

Federal level
    Head   Executive power
      King   *National Fatwah Council*
State level
    Head   Executive power
      Sultan*   *State Mufti*

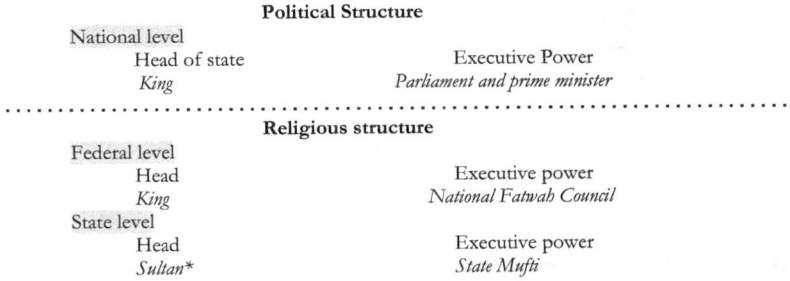

*States with no hereditary sultan take the king as their religious head

Figure 8.1 Diagram of political and religious structures in Malaysia

in the state list of the constitution,[4] including marriage, inheritance, endowments, bequests, violations not governed by federal law[5] and infractions against religion (Kamali, 1997). The constitution stipulates that the *Shariah* courts system and *Shariah* law in Malaysia apply only to Muslim citizens. Malaysians are issued with statutorily required identity cards, which list the citizen's religion (Kamali, 1997). When state-level disputes arise involving both Muslim and non-Muslim parties, the jurisdiction of the Muslim party falls within the *Shariah* courts, and that of the non-Muslims falls within the federal courts (Kamali, 1997).

    The global wave of Islamic revival (Kamali, 1997) seen since the 1970s and 80s, first prompted by the *da'wah* (inviting to Islam) movements, led to several states

4   "1. Except with respect to the Federal Territories of Kuala Lumpur and Labuan, Islamic law and personal and family law of persons professing the religion of Islam, including the Islamic law relating to succession, testate and intestate, betrothal, marriage, divorce, dower, maintenance, adoption, legitimacy guardianship, gifts, partitions and non-charitable trusts; Wakafs and the definition and regulation of charitable and religious endowments, institutions, trusts, charities and charitable institutions operating wholly within the State; Malay customs. Zakat, Fitrah and Baitulmal or similar Islamic religious revenue, mosques or any Islamic public places of worship, creation and punishment of **offences by persons professing the religion of Islam against precepts of that religion** [emphasis added], except in regard to matters included in the Federal List; the constitution, organisation and procedure of [Shariah] courts, which shall have jurisdiction only over person professing the religion of Islam and in respect only of any of the matters included in this paragraph, but shall not have jurisdiction in respect of offences except in so far as conferred by federal law, the control of propagating doctrines and beliefs among persons professing the religion of Islam; the determination of matters of Islamic law and doctrine Malay custom" (Constitution of Malaysia (1957). Ninth schedule, Legislative lists, List II – State list. http://www.commonlii.org/my/legis/const/1957/24.html (Last accessed 9 September 2015)).
5   These include "matrimonial offences, *khalwat* (intimate proximity between a male Muslim and a woman, whether Muslim or non-Muslim, to whom he is not married)" (Kamali, Mohammad Hashim. (2000). *Islamic law in Malaysia: Issues and developments*. Kuala Lumpur: Ilmiah Publishers).

calling for more widespread application of Islamic law in Malaysia. States have also "chosen to exercise their power to create Islamic laws more assertively and have established an increasing number of regulations that are binding on Muslims within their borders" (Shuaib, 2012, p. 91). During the colonial era and following independence, decisions made by *Shariah* courts could be appealed and overruled by civil courts, however, after repeated calls from states to establish a self-contained *Shariah* based legal system, in 1988 a constitutional amendment eliminated the ability to appeal a *Shariah* ruling in the civil courts.[6] The states are able to implement their own interpretation of Islamic law, and the 1988 amendment prevents the federal government from enforcing a uniform Islamic law. There have been attempts, however, to encourage consistency between states through the Ministry of Islamic Development (JAKIM).[7] There have also been suggestions to establish a "grand *mufti*" whose rulings would unite all Muslims of Malaysia (Shuaib, 2012). However, this possibility has not been met with much support, as the states prefer their independence and ability to interpret the Islamic law according to their circumstances.

The contemporary organisation of Islamic authority at the federal and state level in Malaysia

Five national infrastructural features have been identified as being key for considering how Islamic authority in Malaysia is organised at the federal and state levels. These include the constitution, the Department of Islamic Development of Malaysia (JAKIM), the federal courts, the state *Shariah* courts, *muftis* and *fatwah* councils.

i. The Constitution

Federal law in Malaysia is commonly referred to as "secular law", as the remit for legislating according to the *Shariah* is largely limited to the state level *Shariah* courts. However, within the constitution Islam is named as the constitutional religion. Commentators have indicated, therefore, that the federal government could establish a national application of Islamic law, without violating the constitution (Shuaib, 2012). However, as Malaysia is a multi-ethnic, multi-faith society with relatively large Chinese and Indian minorities, and the ruling political party comprises a coalition representing the three largest ethnic groups, the government has articulated no interest in establishing the *Shariah* at the federal level.

---

6   Act A704 Constitution (Amendment) Act (1988). https://www.icrc.org/applic/ihl/ihl-nat.nsf/0/c3dc782c31fa5918c1256a2b004ed898/$FILE/Constitution_en.pdf (Last accessed 15 January 2020).
7   Jabatan Kemajuan Islam Malaysia. (2019). http://www.islam.gov.my/en (Last accessed 15 January 2020).

ii. The Department of Islamic Development of Malaysia (JAKIM)

JAKIM was established in 1997 to enable the development of Islamic institutions and to help standardize the establishment of Islamic law across Malaysia (Shuaib, 2012). JAKIM is responsible for disseminating *fatawah* issued by the National *Fatwah* Council. It also promotes awareness of Islam and its teachings through a web platform, publications as well as an Islamic TV channel.[8] The Department of *Shariah* Judiciary, within JAKIM, was established in 1998[9] to support the infrastructure, development and governance of the *Shariah* courts (Shuaib, 2012) and is headed by the chief *Shariah* judge.

iii. Federal courts and their role in the Malaysian Islamic legal system

National law in Malaysia is developed from statute as well as juridical rulings, where some judges may rely on both common law and Islamic law to arrive at a verdict (Shuaib, 2012). Islamic finance, which initially fell under the jurisdiction of state law, became increasingly important in Malaysia over the past two decades and so had to be regulated by the federal courts (Shuaib, 2012). The federal courts also settle disputes relating to freedom of religion in cases where there may have been violations of Muslims' rights.

An additional layer of complexity emerges in the role of the federal courts within the federal territories that comprise Kuala Lumpur, Putrajaya, and Labuan. These constitute Malaysia's capital and do not form a state; rather, they fall directly under the jurisdiction of the federal government and federal courts. If there are disputes relating to Islamic law in the federal territories, they are arbitrated not in a *Shariah* court but within the federal courts (Shuaib, 2012).

iv. State Shariah *courts and their role in the Malaysian Islamic legal system*

As stated above, the constitution allows states to adjudicate according to Islamic law within a *Shariah* court system. The jurisdiction of the state *Shariah* courts includes religious observance, such as *Zakat* (giving of charity); family law, such marriage and divorce and personal laws, such as inheritance. Additionally, *Shariah* courts have the legal power to implement Islamic criminal law (Shuaib, 2012). Although criminal law is largely under the federal system, limited powers have been granted to the *Shariah* courts to enforce Islamic criminal law for "offences by persons professing the religion of Islam against precepts of that religion".[10] The classification of these offences is important for biomedical research, as they

---

8   Jabatan Kemajuan Islam Malaysia. (2017). WebTV Rasmi. http://www.tvjakim.my (Last accessed 28 March 2020).
9   JKSM. (2019). Official website: Department of Syariah Judiciary Malaysia. http://www.jksm.gov.my/index.php/ms (Last accessed 15 January 2020).
10 Constitution of Malaysia (1957). Ninth schedule, Legislative lists, List II – State list. http://www.commonlii.org/my/legis/const/1957/24.html (Last accessed 15 January 2020).

concern views about homosexuality, transsexuality and sexual relations out of wedlock (Shuaib, 2012). More recently, states that hold a "conservative" interpretation (Kamali, 1997, pp. 154, 178) of Islam and Islamic law have tried to implement *Hudud* law (capital punishment according to Islamic law), however, this has been resisted at the federal level (Kamali, 1997).

v. Muftis, fatawah *and* fatwah *councils – a parallel Islamic legal system*

Within Malaysia's legislative process, parallel to the federal and *Shariah* courts, is an alternate system for constructing and ratifying laws through a body of *muftis* or religious legal scholars. Each state has a *mufti*, commonly appointed by the sultan or by the king in the federal territories, who can issue *fatawah* or legal rulings based on Islamic law. Such *fatawah* can also be issued by the state or federal *fatwah* committees, which are groups of religious legal scholars. The process of appointing a *mufti* is opaque, and studies have shown that the qualifications and experience of *muftis* within Malaysia are very diverse (Shuaib, 2012). The state *mufti* acts as the head of the state *fatwah* council. When a *mufti* or the council issue a *fatwah*, in order for it to become state law, it is considered by the National *Fatwah* Council and, once approved, it is accepted by the state sultan. Once the state sultan accepts a *fatwah*, it is binding and is applied by the *Shariah* courts (Shuaib, 2012). As mentioned above, with each state having its own *mufti* and *fatwah* council, which can interpret Islamic law differently, there has been a variation in what is considered to be the Islamic legal opinion in Malaysia.

Malaysia as a suitable site for this study

Studies have highlighted that Malaysia's multicultural society "welcomes freedom of expression and religious views" (Imam et al., 2009, p. 89). Imam et al. (2009) explain that, whilst "increasing numbers of Malays are becoming more religious", there are many who are not (p. 89). The resulting "ideological dichotomy" is "reflected in the fact that [the] interpretation of Islam in Malaysia in relatively liberal in contrast to the popular conception of Islamic nations" (Imam et al., 2009, p. 89). Malaysia is a rare example of successful cooperation between "proponents of strict secularisation and Islamic factions within the country" (Imam et al., 2009, p. 89). This is seen in aspects of Malaysian society, such as business and lifestyle, where *Shariah* compliance is sought within the overall national commitment to modernise. Such a commitment to balancing *Shariah* compliance and modernisation is now being seen within the sciences (Setia, 2007).

Malaysia, with its recent investment in research ethics committees and guidelines,[11] its Muslim majority and its state level implementation of Islamic law, was a suitable case study for this research. Malaysia presented an ideal environment to enable an exploration of how ethical concepts are understood and

---

11 Malaysia Medical Research and Ethics Committee (MREC). http://nih.gov.my/web/mrec/ (Last accessed 15 January 2020).

implemented, and how Islam influences ethico-legal decision-making within biomedical research. Within Malaysia, interviews were conducted in the capital city, Kuala Lumpur, the more religiously "conservative" (Kamali, 1997, pp. 154, 178) northeast coast state, Kelantan, and the northwest state Penang. These areas were selected to capture views in different states with differing religo-political landscapes.

Iran: A brief historical and contemporary overview of the socioeconomic and religio-ethnic context

The Islamic Republic of Iran, a country in Asia straddled by the Persian Gulf and the Caspian Sea with a population of approximately 63 million (Delvoie & Ansari, 2001), is a Muslim majority country (99%).[12] With the fourth largest oil reserves and second largest reserves of natural gas (Delvoie & Ansari, 2001), Iran has been in the geopolitical spotlight for decades. Since antiquity, in fact, Iran has held an important strategic place in the historical narrative of civilisations. Alongside its colourful ancient and contemporary political history, Iran is a myriad of religious and intellectual movements and ideas (Axworthy, 2010, pp. 1–30). Iran has found a unique place in the Muslim world as the only Islamic state, which was formed after the 1979 revolution. Since the revolution there has been a commitment to incorporate Islamic values within the modern state and to place Muslim scholars at the centre of national legislation (Gheissair et al., 2009, pp. 105–20). Iran is a country of "paradoxes", where some scholars have commented that, despite the support for the revolution and subsequent adoption of Islamic law within the state, only 1.4 percent of the population attend Friday prayers (Axworthy, 2010, p. xiii). There is repeated condemnation of materialism and "Western" values, yet contemporary Iranian society aspires to the enhancements offered by cosmetic surgery (Ansari, 2014, p. 6), with the demand for such interventions increasing at an exponential rate. For this research, it was deemed important, therefore, to assess the influence of personal religious convictions versus the laws and ideologies implemented at the state level when examining ethical decision-making in the healthcare research context within Iran.

Iran's history is important for providing context, but also for shedding light on the experiences of Iranians. Ansari (2014) suggests that Iran's past is used as a political tool to reshape the present and future, where governments select carefully what they choose to remember, and also what they forget. It is important, therefore, to explore Iran's relationship with its past in order to understand current trends and future projections.

12 Pew Research Forum (2009). Mapping the global Muslim population. http://www.pewforum.org/2009/10/07/mapping-the-global-muslim-population (Last accessed 15 January 2020).

The arrival of Islam in Iran – The Arab conquest and the fall of the Sasanian empire

Pre-Islamic Iran was ruled by a Sasanian monarchy, and the prevailing religion was Zoroastrianism (Axworthy, 2010, pp. 1–30). However, the Sasanian dynasty suffered heavy military losses during the reign of Khosraw II, which provided Arab conquerors a key victory in Qadesiyya in 637 AD (Axworthy, 2010, pp. 1–30), and the capture of the whole of Mesopotamia soon followed. Although Arab rulers and Islam replaced the Sasanian monarchy and Zoroastrian faith, the culture and language of the Persians survived and even flourished. Researchers suggest that Modern Persian is relatively unchanged since the 11th century (Axworthy, 2010, pp. 31–66). Poetry and literature is preserved deeply within the conscience and culture of modern Iranian society, with Firdausi's *Shahnameh* being considered a masterpiece and integral to the Iranian identity. The epic poem explores the critical transition in Iran's history from the Sasanian Monarchy and Zoroastrian faith to the Arab Muslim conquest and the predominance of Islam. That Iranians consider Firdausi's epic a national treasure, with its central themes exploring a key historical transition, providing provides insight into the complex role of religion and state authority in Iran (Ansari, 2014, pp. 11–8).

When the Arabs conquered Persia, the Zoroastrians were afforded a similar respect by the Muslims as offered to the Christians and Jews (people of the book), where they were free to follow their faiths if they paid the necessary tax (*jizyah*) to the state (Axworthy, 2010, pp. 67–120). The wealthy families had an economic interest, therefore, in converting to Islam, while those from lower socioeconomic groups remained non-Muslim for many centuries (Axworthy, 2010, pp. 67–120). The period of transition was wrought with violence, however, including the murder of Zoroastrian priests and destruction of temples. Overall, historians suggest that the Iranian people benefitted from the replacement of an aristocracy, which heavily taxed its subjects, by a more egalitarian society established through Muslim rule, where there was a greater emphasis on serving the poor (Axworthy, 2010, pp. 67–120).

The origins of Shi'ism *and establishment of a* Shi'i *politico-legal system*

One of the most important features of Iran's history is the establishment of *Shi'i* Islam and the *Shi'i* state. The *Shi'i* school gained political recognition when the Safavid dynasty came to power in the late 15th century. Ismaili *Shi'ism* was adopted by the ruling elite in Iran, establishing a *Shi'i* state. Iranian *Shi'i* philosophy and theology is heavily influenced by the *Mu'tazilis*, who emphasised free will and the role of reason in the interpretation of the *Qur'an* and *Hadith* (Winter, 2008, pp. 1–14; see also Chapter 1). Tremayne (2009) reports that *Shi'i* scholars' reliance on reason (*ijtihad*) to interpret the *Qur'an*, a practice she describes as "unique to the *Shia* sect" (Tremayne, 2009, p. 147) has led to the development of a more fluid religious interpretation within the *Shi'i* legal system, in comparison to the *Sunni* system, which is still visible in Iran today (Tremayne, 2009, pp. 144–63).

Establishment of the Islamic Republic of Iran

Since their inception, the *Shia* have considered themselves "the underdogs, the disposed, those always betrayed and humiliated by the powerful and unrighteous" (Axworthy, 2010, p. 127). Such sentiments have remained within the Iranian psyche to this day, and they extend beyond the *Sunni* world to Western nations, such as the US. Feelings of oppression and the tendency to recoil from corrupt authority led to the national fervour that ignited the revolution in 1979 (Axworthy, 2010, pp. 221–58). The Iran-Iraq War, which followed the revolution, was fuelled by Saddam Hossein's anti-*Shia* sentiment and supported by *Sunni* states, such as Saudi Arabia. Western states sided with Iraq, fuelling Iran's national feelings of isolation, betrayal and persecution.

Ruhollah Khomeini, who was a descendent of the Prophet Muhammad, grew in popularity as a "*marja*", or one to be followed, by an increasing number of students who attended his lectures on ethics in the early 1960s (Axworthy, 2010, pp. 221–58). Returning from exile in 1979, he was considered "the focal point of the hopes of a whole nation" (Axworthy, 2010, p. 259). Reports suggest that as he passed euphoric crowds, they addressed him as "*Oh Imam*" (Axworthy, 2010, p. 260). The title of *Imam* is a significant one in *Shia* theology, and it strengthened Khomeini's leadership. The people thus transferred authority from a monarchy to a religious Ayatollah. Historians consider the revolution as not simply a religious one; rather, it emerged as a result of economic frustrations, corruption and oppression (Axworthy, 2010, pp. 259–82). Khomeini's charisma, combined with a collective *Shi'i* sentiment for political change and the transfer of authority to a theocracy, led to what was, even if briefly, "a people's revolution" (Axworthy, 2010, p. 261), which united disparate factions for a common purpose. The Islamic revivalist movement in Iran, as seen in Malaysia, also reflected the more widespread Islamisation seen in the Muslim world during the 1970s and 80s (Entessar, 1988).

The contemporary organisation of Islamic authority in Iran

The following details the infrastructural organisation of Islamic authority in Iran, including the constitution, the Supreme Leader, the Council of Guardians, the President and Parliament, and the judiciary.

i. The Constitution

For Khomeini and those who supported the revolution, the Shah's monarchy represented corruption and excessive foreign influence within its judicial system (Entessar, 1988). Once in power, Khomeini initiated the replacement of a Eurocentric "man-made" legal system to one that relied on "God-given laws" (Entessar, 1988). He emphasised that the establishment of the *Shariah* would provide a just system for the people. He therefore extended the role of Muslim scholars beyond offering religious advice to that of establishing an Islamic government

(Entessar, 1988). Articles 1 and 2 of the Iranian Constitution reflect this shift in authority.[13] Article 2[14] further emphasises the reliance on "Divine Will" (Entessar, 1988) and the role of scholars in determining God's will. The constitution thus cements the authority of the Supreme Leader, who is the religious/spiritual head, and the role of other Muslim scholars (*muftis*), who through their religious training have sole authority to interpret the primary sources and issue legal rulings.

ii. The Supreme Leader

The Iranian Constitution of 1979 entrusted highest politico-legal power to the Supreme Leader. The post was initially held by Ayatollah Khomeini, and after his death it passed over to Ayatollah Khamenei. The Constitution emphasises the Twelver *Shi'ism* (the dominant sect in Iran) belief that, in the absence of the Twelfth *Imam* (twelfth descendent of Ali), all political and legal power derives from the Supreme Leader (Entessar, 1988).

iii. The Council of Guardians

Article 4 of the Constitution banned all laws that were considered against the *Shariah* and placed the highest legal authority at the level of the Council of Guardians – a body of jurists considered sufficiently qualified in the Islamic sciences.[15] The Council has the legal authority to veto laws passed by the parliament

13 "The form of government of Iran is that of an Islamic Republic, endorsed by the people of Iran on the basis of their longstanding belief in the sovereignty of truth and Qur'anic justice … through the affirmative vote of a majority of 98.2% of eligible voters, held after the victorious Islamic Revolution led by the eminent marji' al-taqlid, Ayatullah al-Uzma Imam Khumayni." (Constitution of the Islamic Republic of Iran. (1979). https://www.refworld.org/docid/3ae6b56710.html (Last accessed 28 March 2020)).

14 "The Islamic Republic is a system based on belief in: (1.) The One God (as stated in the phrase 'There is no god except Allah'), His exclusive sovereignty and the right to legislate, and the necessity of submission to His commands; (2.) Divine revelation and its fundamental role in setting forth the laws; (3.) the return to God in the Hereafter, and the constructive role of this belief in the course of man's ascent towards God; (4.) the justice of God in creation and legislation; (5.) continuous leadership (imamah) and perpetual guidance, and its fundamental role in ensuring the uninterrupted process of the revolution of Islam; (6.) the exalted dignity and value of man, and his freedom coupled with responsibility before God; in which equity, justice, political, economic, social, and cultural independence, and national solidarity are secured by recourse to: (i.) continuous ijtihad of the fuqaha' possessing necessary qualifications, exercised on the basis of the Qur'an and the Sunnah of the Ma'sumun, upon all of whom be peace; (ii.) sciences and arts and the most advanced results of human experience, together with the effort to advance them further; (iii.) negation of all forms of oppression, both the infliction of and the submission to it, and of dominance, both its imposition and its acceptance" (Constitution of the Islamic Republic of Iran. (1979). https://www.refworld.org/docid/3ae6b56710.html (Last accessed 28 March 2020)).

15 "Article 4: All civil, penal financial, economic, administrative, cultural, military, political, and other laws and regulations must be based on Islamic criteria. This principle applies absolutely and generally to all articles of the Constitution as well as to all other

(Entessar, 1988). It "informed the Supreme Judicial Council on April 16, 1981 that constitutionally only the Council of Guardians has the authority to pass final judgment on the propriety of any new law or the validity of any pre-revolutionary legislation" (Entessar, 1988, p. 95).

iv. The President and Parliament

Although the Supreme Leader and Guardian Council are unelected, the election of the president and parliamentary positions are growing in importance. The democratic process does not supersede the Islamic system established through the supreme leader and Guardian Council; however, it does determine the distribution of political power in the 31 provinces, and it influences policymaking (Gheissair et al., 2009, pp. 23–50). Political commentators suggest that, although the Iranian constitution "vests sovereignty in God" (Gheissair et al., 2009, p. vi) and "state behaviour in Iran does not normatively reflect, democratic values" (Gheissair et al., 2009, p. vi), there are growing tensions at the grassroots level, with increasing political influence pressed by "civil society activism and elections to voice social and political demands" (Gheissair et al., 2009, p. vi).

The election of President Khatami in 1997 marked a shift in Iranian politics. Khatami was aware of growing public frustration, especially amongst young people, with the theocratic regime and extra-judicial violence and killing. Axworthy (2010) suggests that Khatami pushed for reforms in order to save the Islamic Republic, however, his reforms were blocked (pp. 259–82). Historians suggest that the veto of Khatami's reforms led to the regime's further unpopularity and disillusionment with the Islamic leadership, which was reflected in the drop in attendance of Friday prayers (Axworthy, 2010, p. xiii). Khatami's presidency highlighted a schism in the Iranian public's expectations – those committed to hard-line *Shi'i* Islam hoped for a more religiously conservative government reflected in the subsequent election of Ahmedinijad, whereas others hoped for a more secular government.

President Rouhani's election in 2013 and subsequent policies responded to Khatami's anxieties and reflected Iran's struggle to retain a theocracy whilst re-establishing ties with the rest of the world. The latter is of particular importance to the younger population in Iran who are increasingly frustrated with international sanctions and global suspicions of Iran and Iranian people.[16] Rouhani's reputation within the Council of Guardians and his awareness of the global climate has made him popular with both religiously conservative factions and those seeking a more secular government (Delvoie & Ansari, 2001). His policies reflect the growing

laws and regulations, and the fuqaha' of the Guardian Council are judges in this matter." (Constitution of the Islamic Republic of Iran. (1979). https://www.refworld.org/docid/3ae6b56710.html (Last accessed 28 March 2020)).

16 In his 2002 State of the Union Address to Congress, President George W. Bush labelled Iran as one of that states that constituted "the Axis of Evil" (Office of the Press Secretary. (2002). President delivers State of the Union address. http://georgew bush-whitehouse.archives.gov/news/releases/2002/01/20020129-11.html).

power of civil society and the emerging challenges of how Iran will manage to retain its *Shi'i* theocracy whilst meeting the demands of a rapidly evolving populace calling for democracy (Delvoie & Ansari, 2001).

v. The judiciary

All Iranian courts follow the *Shariah*, and the Supreme Leader appoints the Chief Justice. The judges in every court must be versed in *Shia* jurisprudence or undergo necessary training before taking up judicial positions.[17] Iran has a centralised system of law through the Supreme Judicial Council (Entessar, 1988), which ensures there is no variation in the application of the penal code.

Overall, therefore, the Supreme Leader has the widest mandate in the running of the state and the issuing of legal edicts. The Guardian Council is afforded the function of an "upper house" (Mir-Hosseini, 2010, pp. 319–72), which can veto parliamentary laws that are deemed non-*Shariah* compliant and issue *fatawah* on issues brought to its attention. The Parliament is able to ratify laws, and the courts are able to issue rulings based on the cases that are presented to them. Islamic law, and more specifically *Shi'i* law, pervades throughout the Iranian politico-legal system. An empirical study was considered suitable to help elucidate the impact of Islam's politico-legal role within the biomedical research context in Iran.

Iran as a suitable site for this study

Although there has been little work within the *Sunni* Muslim tradition dealing with the ethical challenges posed by biomedical research, the *Shia* tradition, primarily based in Iran, displays a burgeoning scholarly input within this field. The *Shia* tradition focuses not on the consensus (*Ijma*) of scholars, but rather on independent scholarly reasoning (*Ijtihad*) (Zali et al., 2002). There have been rapid efforts within Iran to not only address the ethical challenges posed by emerging technologies, but also challenges posed by clinical trials and externally sponsored research (Larijani et al., 2006).

Larijani et al. (2005) have described the method through which Islamic values are considered within the context of bioethics:

> In the Islamic Republic of Iran, ethical issues are discussed among physicians, legal experts and religious scholars. The principles of bioethics and solutions to ethical problems are therefore derived from the Islamic legal rulings. They are updated in the light of the Holy Quran, the traditions of the Prophet of Islam (Peace Be Upon Him), the consensus of scholars, and human wisdom or intellect.
>
> (p. 1063)

17 Omar Sial. (2006). A guide to the legal system of the Islamic Republic of Iran. https://www.nyulawglobal.org/globalex/Iran.html (Last accessed 28 March 2020).

Thus, it was deemed important to evaluate the process of textual and contextual consultation in such a setting as well as to review how subsequent guidelines also impact practice at the individual researcher level.

Bioethical discourse has a long history in Iran, with scholars such as Ibn Sina writing about the importance ethico-legal considerations in medicine in the tenth century (Sachedina, 2009, p. 197). Since then, the teaching and practising of bioethics has been emphasised greatly in Iran (Larijani & Zahedi, 2008). Contemporary commitments to bioethics legislation are highlighted in the development of the National Committee of Medical Research Ethics in 1997 (Zahedi et al., 2008) and the subsequent establishment of local institutional review boards. In 2000, the Ministry of Health and Medical Education (MOHME) authored and ratified into law the National Code of Ethics. Its 26 articles have been described as being coherent with both "international declarations and Islamic codes" (Zahedi et al., 2008, p. 631).

There is paucity of published research on qualitative analyses of the impact of such structures and guidelines on the ethical decision-making of researchers and research ethics committees in Iran. With its historical and contemporary ethico-legal narrative, Iran presented a unique opportunity to explore in depth the Islamic influence on biomedical research ethics at the state, institutional and individual levels.

Thus, Malaysia and Iran, with their recent investment in biomedical research and research ethics infrastructure as well as their complex histories and the role of religion, presented ideal locations for the exploration of the role of Islam in the ethical decision-making of researchers, RECs and guideline developers in the biomedical research context.

Why are qualitative methods a suitable tool of empirical investigation for this research?

The literature review revealed that little is known about Muslim researchers, researchers who work with Muslim participants and the types of questions and problems they face. Qualitative methods, such as in-depth interviews, are "ideal for exploring topics where little is known", and they enable an understanding of "complex situations, gaining insight into phenomena, constructing themes to explain phenomena, and ultimately fostering deep understanding of the phenomena" (Smith et al., 2011, p. 3). It is a suitable method for understanding meaning and context, particularly where little work has been done previously.

Although quantitative methods, such as questionnaires, can be employed to collate researchers' views on the utility of guidelines or the types of problems they face, such tools rely on existing data in order to construct appropriate questions. The purpose of this study is to explore the distinct problems faced by Muslims researchers, ethics committee members and those who work within a Muslim context. The exploration of complex issues, such as the influence of cultural and religious factors on ethical decision-making in the research context, would be extremely difficult with pre-defined quantitative methods (Silverman, 2013, pp. 5–

15). Qualitative methods provide a means of developing an initial insight into phenomena, generating new hypotheses and understanding complex situations, which can then be employed to construct and enhance quantitative tools of investigation (Green et al., 2013, pp. 1–33). Qualitative methods, therefore, are a more suitable means of approaching the question than, for example, a survey.

Why use semi-structured interviews for data collection and a case study method to explore themes?

Case study methodology

As the focus of this study was to understand ethical decision-making within the contexts in which researchers reside, a case study method provided an ideal means of exploring themes and their interactions. Crowe et al. (2011) explain: "the case study approach is particularly useful to employ when there is a need to obtain an in-depth appreciation of an issue, event or phenomenon of interest, in its natural real-life context". As researchers' decision-making is multifaceted and their context multi-layered, an in-depth case study provided an ideal means of disentangling these relevant factors and enabling a reflection on their interactions, impact and influences. The political, socioeconomic and religio-cultural context within which researchers make ethical decisions needed to be understood, and a case-study approach allowed an exploration of these themes.

The type of case study employed was a "collective case study", as described by Stake (2000), "where a number of cases are studied to investigate some general phenomenon" (pp. 437–8). In this study, the cases of Malaysia and Iran were used together to analyse the influence of Islam on biomedical research ethics. The case studies of Iran and Malaysia were, therefore, considered conceptually linked, as they were both being employed to investigate the phenomenon of Islam's influence on biomedical research ethics (Crowe et al., 2011). The data for the countries are therefore presented as cross-cutting and thematically arranged, rather than case-by-case. This was done to emphasise that the focus of this study is the role of Islam in the decision-making of researchers, REC members and scholars, and not simply how research ethics is done in the two countries. It was also to enable an analysis of similarities between the two countries and to outline differences. A cross-cutting approach also prevented repetition in the reporting of the analysis, especially as early interviews in Iran revealed that similar themes were found to those analysed in Malaysia. Finally, the methodological aim of this study was not to artificially separate "Islam" by the national boundaries of the two countries; rather, this study sought to explore what can collectively be learnt from the two case study sites about what "Islam" is in the biomedical research context and how "Islam" influences research ethics. Of course, it is important to acknowledge here that the participants' contexts may influence their views on the "what" and "how" as they pertain to Islam and biomedical research ethics. Other participants from other countries may have differing views. Thus, the choice and number of sites may limit the generalizability of the research findings and, in particular, what can be generalised about Islam. These limitations will be further elaborated upon later in this chapter.

By choosing a "collective case study" and aiming to present the two cases of Iran and Malaysia as cross-cutting, the implications for the analysis were that the earlier interviews in Iran had to be carefully analysed in order to determine whether it was possible to present the two countries or cases together. If the interview guide developed for interviews in Malaysia was deemed unsuitable, or if very different themes emerged in Iran, then the study would have required that the two countries be treated as separate cases, both in the analysis and presentation of the data. However, after conducting three to four interviews in Iran and completing a preliminary analysis of the transcripts, I found that there were similar themes to those encountered in Malaysia. This meant that a cross-cutting presentation was suitable for the study.

The cases in both Malaysia and Iran were inevitably bounded by the time period spent in the two sites, careful reading and analysis of the literature about the two cases, including relevant historical and geopolitical factors, in order to situate the research around the views of biomedical researchers, REC members, guideline developers and scholars. The analysis was, therefore, limited to the views of these participants and the particular time period of the research, which, in turn, also limits the generalizability of the findings. However, as the focus of this study was to investigate the influence of Islam on biomedical research, it was deemed suitable to bound the study to this group. Future work may consider extending the cases to include other potential stakeholders, such as research participants, research funders and political figures.

I was also keen to interview participants at differing institutions and from different cities in the two countries, as the background reading revealed Islam's very different role in the different regions of Malaysia, for example. The latter did influence the data collection and analysis, as it was important to familiarise myself with the background of the different regions in the two countries in order to understand the responses of participants and probe appropriately. During the analysis it was important to consider the region within which participants were based in order to enable appropriate comparison, analysis and understanding of their views.

Semi-structured interviews

Green et al. (2013) describe the interview as "a conversation that is directed, more or less, towards the researcher's particular needs for data" (p. 95). As I wanted to explore themes arising from the literature, such as genetic research and tissue storage, these were the particular topics explored in the interviews (see the Appendix for the draft interview guide). However, it was important to ensure that the participants' also had the opportunity to describe and explain their unique experiences and the distinct ethical problems they faced. Therefore, a semi-structured interview method was used, which combined open discussion with a more directed discussion of pre-existing topics, followed by the extraction of themes from participants' responses to further probe their reasoning and to explore emerging topics. As one of the objectives of the study was to investigate whether and how people's personal religious beliefs impacted their understanding and approaches to biomedical research ethics, the semi-structured interview presented the ideal means of probing and also challenging participants' views to better understand their reasoning and experiences.

Throughout the study I consulted the literature and other sources of information, such as policy documents, websites, guidelines and laws at regional, national and district levels, to inform the interview guide, complement the data obtained from interviews and supplement the data analysis and discussion. The review of the literature and documentation had been useful in yielding information about the existing ethico-legal infrastructures, health research priorities and processes in Iran and Malaysia, which enabled appropriate probing within the interviews when such factors were mentioned.

Another advantage of using interviews over other qualitative methods, such as focus groups, was that the nature of this study and its exploration of people's individual faith required a one-to-one discussion, the opportunity for participants to privately reflect and respond to questions and confidential probing where such a process would be less likely to cause discomfort. In both Malaysia and Iran, the historical and contemporary role and authority of Islam is sensitive and complex. Such complexity required a methodology that ensured the confidentiality of participants and was sensitive to their needs.

Why was the framework approach a suitable method of analysis?

A framework approach was used because it has been described as a flexible method of analysis that allows for both inductive and deductive contributions to analysis. Concepts and themes from the literature and guideline review were used as pre-existing theoretical constructs during the analysis of the data (deductive analysis), alongside an inductive approach, whereby themes were identified directly from the qualitative data before revisiting the literature (Gale et al., 2013). As this study focuses on describing and analysing the reasons and processes underlying decision-making in the context of specific ethical questions, grounded theory, with its focus on theory development, rather than the description of social processes (Smith et al., 2011), was not an appropriate method for this research. A framework analysis, by contrast, is suitable for "identify[ing] commonalities and differences in qualitative data, before focusing on relationships between different parts of the data, thereby seeking to draw descriptive and/or explanatory conclusions clustered around themes" (Gale et al., 2013, p. 2). This method also has the advantage that, although in-depth analysis can take place across the entire dataset, the process of coding and charting ensures that the views of each participant remain connected within a matrix (Gale et al., 2013). The data analysis in this study employed the thematic framework analysis method devised by Ritchie and Lewis (2003). A detailed account of the application of the framework analysis is described in subsequent sections of this chapter.

Data sources and types

1 Semi-structured interviews were carried out in order to address the study aims of gaining an understanding of participants' views on the types of ethical questions they encounter, how they address these questions, and the role of personal faith and Islamic normative sources in the characterisation and response to ethical questions.

2 A quantitative religiosity survey developed by Huber and Huber (2012), which has been used in over 100 studies in 25 different countries involving over 100,000 participants (Huber & Huber, 2012),[18] was used to optimise recruitment of Muslim participants in Malaysia by attempting to capture the views of a mixture of religious and non-religious participants. In Iran this was not possible, as the inclusion of a "religiosity survey" was considered inappropriate by my local contact. The explanation given was that "expressed religiosity" is a politically sensitive issue in Iran, and it would make participants uncomfortable and could even bias their responses within the interview. Being mindful of such potential challenges, I decided the survey was not appropriate in Iran. During the interviews in Iran, participants were able to express their views about the role of religion, both positive and negative, and they were forthcoming about their own religiosity/irreligiosity, so the absence of the survey did not affect my ability to gather rich and varied accounts within the interviews.

3 Sociodemographic data were collected for each participant to capture views from a range of ages, genders, research experience levels and locations.

4 Direct observation was also used throughout the study period to familiarize myself with the different contexts and to inform my interview style, e.g., noticing non-verbal cues, such as anxiety/uncertainty, in order to alter questioning and probing.

5 Detailed field notes were also kept daily to reflect on each of the interviews and what was being learnt regarding the socio-political and religious contexts whilst spending time in the two countries.

Study visits

Each site was visited to ensure adequate time for familiarisation with the context, recruitment of eligible participants and data collection. The placement in Malaysia was for ten weeks from mid-November 2014 to January 2015. The placement in Iran was for four weeks between the end of April and the end of May 2015. The period of time spent in Iran was shorter partly due to pragmatism, as the visa issued was for one month, but also because recruitment of participants was easier. Fewer participants were interviewed due to there being a scarcity of non-Muslim researchers in Iran, and data saturation was reached.

---

18 The authors kindly provided a version of the questionnaire that they specifically use for Muslim participants.

Sampling strategy for research participants

Given the aim of the study, the following types of key stakeholders were identified as important and included in recruitment:

- Researchers, either principle investigators or fieldworkers (Muslim and non-Muslim)
- REC members (Muslim and non-Muslim)
- Guideline developers (Muslim and non-Muslim)
- Islamic scholars involved in the biomedical research context, either as a guideline author/consultant or as a member of a REC or scholarly *fatwah* council.

The rationale for sampling these four types of interviewees was because they constitute the four groups most likely to be able to provide insight into the role of Islam in biomedical research practice.

The rationale for interviewing diverse actors at multiple levels of research prioritisation, design and implementation was to allow for an assessment of the multiple relevant perspectives within biomedical research in the different contexts. It was also a means by which the complex interaction of the different players and the various cultural and religious contexts could be analysed.

The research participants were drawn from the three/four settings within each country, with the requirement that they will have had some experience of clinical research, either through consultation (e.g., Muslim scholars) or direct experience (researchers and principle investigators of trials). A purposive sampling method was employed to capture a range of experiences.

For the tiers of participants (listed above), I attempted to include both Muslim and non-Muslim participants in Malaysia. This was to allow an assessment of how the individuals' beliefs impacted both the consultative and practical stages of biomedical research guideline production, involvement in RECs as well personal practical deliberations when carrying out research. This was not possible in Iran, as there are too few non-Muslim researchers. The semi-structured interview method employed focused on in-depth data gathering per participant, rather than on recruiting large samples (Smith et al., 2011).

In this empirical study "Islamic scholars", for the purposes of participant recruitment, were defined as individuals who had received formal training in the Islamic sciences and had graduated having been conferred the recognition of either *Alim* (an expert in Islamic law and theology) or *mufti* (one who has training and expertise in issuing legal edicts) or *Faqih* (a jurist). It did not include individuals who lead the community in prayer (*Imaam*) unless the individual also carried one or more of the aforementioned qualifications. Although many of the participants in Malaysia and Iran, who were primarily trained in the biomedical sciences, had extensive knowledge of the Islamic sciences, very few had undertaken formal Islamic studies training. The literature refers to those with formal training in the Islamic sciences as Islamic scholars, and the latter are those who are given such an authority by lay Muslims (Padela, 2013a). This definition was used to identify and recruit "Islamic scholars". Islamic scholars were approached who had previously had some involvement in biomedical research, either through an institutional REC, during the process of guideline development or as a member of a scholarly *fatwah* council/institution that had been involved in considering biomedical research issues.

Data collection in Malaysia

Thirty-eight interviews were conducted in Malaysia. This number was based on my being able to interview a sufficient number of suitable individuals within each of the participant categories, such that data saturation was reached, i.e., until a point was reached beyond which it was judged the addition of new themes was unlikely. One interview was conducted via Skype with two participants who were keen to participate in the study, but who had been unavailable during my visit. Although data saturation had been reached prior to this interview, I felt that, given the participants' interest in the study, it would be valuable to include their contributions. The case study participants were from three different states (Kuala Lumpur, Penang and Kelantan) and eight institutions, including state and private universities and state ministries, such as the Malaysia Medical Council and the Institute of Islamic Understanding (IKIM). A full list of institutions is not provided here, as many of the participants requested that their institutions not be named at all in study publications. In order to respect their requests and to main confidentiality, I have not included institutional affiliations in any of the tables, quotes or narrative within this volume.

For interviews in Malaysia, 50 potential participants were identified via web searches of institutional websites, with the advice of Professor Lokman Saim and through suggestions from interview participants (snowball sampling). Twenty-five researchers, ten REC members, eight guideline developers and seven Islamic scholars were identified as potentially suitable for the study. Of these, 39 replied to my initial email. A follow-up email was sent to all other participants; however, no reply was received from 11 individuals (three researchers, two REC members, two guideline developers and four Islamic scholars). Of the 39 replies, only one participant (a REC member) did not answer subsequent emails and was unavailable for interview.

See Table 8.1 for a profile of the Malaysia participants, including gender, age, researcher status (Y/N), REC member status (Y/N), guideline developer status (Y/N), Islamic scholar status (Y/N), and informal training in the Islamic sciences (Y/N). As can be seen from the table, many of the participants had multiple roles and responsibilities, such that the interviews were incredibly rich.

Of the 38 interviews, 33 were conducted in university offices or hospital clinics, and only I was present with the participant. Four of the interviews were carried out in public cafés, which were chosen by the participants as more convenient. Although there were other people in the café, the participant was comfortable that the interview was conducted privately. One interview was carried out over Skype with two participants (Participants 38a & b). Both participants were keen to be interviewed together, as they were working on similar projects and wanted to share their insights jointly.

Data collection in Iran

Eighteen interviews were conducted in Iran. This number was based on my being able to interview a sufficient number of suitable individuals within each of the participant categories, such that data saturation was reached. One interview was conducted via Skype with a participant who was keen to participate in the study but was unavailable during my visit. Although data saturation had been reached prior to this interview, I felt that, given the participant's interest in the study, it would be valuable to include their contribution. The case study participants were from four different cities (Tehran, Qum, Isfahan and Shiraz) and five different institutions and state ministries, including the Ministry of Health and Medical Education (MOHME) and the Medical Ethics and Medical History Research Centre (MEHRC). A full list of institutions is not provided here, as many of the participants requested that their institutions not be named at all in study publications. In order to respect their requests and to maintain confidentiality, I have not included institutional affiliations in any of the tables, quotes or narrative within this volume.

As only Muslim participants were identified for the interviews in Iran, 25 potential participants were identified via web searches of institutional websites, with the advice of Dr. Ehsan Shamsi and through suggestions from interview participants (snowball sampling). Nine researchers, seven REC members, five guideline developers and four Islamic scholars were identified as potentially suitable for the study. As I was only able to make contact with potential participants once I reached Iran, I had to send the initial emails soon after my arrival and received positive responses from 20 people. Two of the potential participants (one scholar and one guideline developer), however, were subsequently unavailable for interview. I did not receive responses from five individuals (two researchers, one REC member and two Islamic scholars).

See Table 8.2 for a profile of the Iran participants, including gender, age, researcher status (Y/N), REC member status (Y/N), guideline developer status (Y/N), Islamic scholar status (Y/N), and informal training in the Islamic sciences (Y/N). As can be seen from the table, many of the participants had multiple roles and responsibilities, which produced incredibly rich interviews.

All of the interviews in Iran were conducted in university offices or hospital clinics. Only two interviews were conducted with a translator present. All other interviews were carried out privately. Translators were asked to keep details of the interviews private, and the participants were comfortable with the translator being present.

Table 8.1 Malaysia participant profile, including gender (male/female), age, researcher (Y/N), REC member (Y/N), guideline developer (Y/N), Islamic scholar (Y/N), and informal training in the Islamic sciences (Y/N)

Participant number	Gender (Male/Female)	Age	Muslim	Researcher	REC member	Guideline author	Islamic scholar	Informal training in Islamic sciences
1	M	56	Y	Y	Y	N	N	Y
2	M	39	Y	Y	Y	N	N	N
3	M	42	N	Y	Y	N	N	N
4	M	65	N	Y	Y	Y	N	N
5	M	55	Y	Y	N	N	N	Y
6	M	64	Y	Y	Y	Y	N	Y
7	M	53	Y	Y	Y	Y	N	N
8	F	32	N	Y	N	N	N	N
9	M	47	N	Y	N	N	N	N
10	M	35	Y	Y	Y	N	N	Y
11	M	50	Y	Y	N	N	N	N
12	F	32	Y	Y	N	N	N	N
13	F	53	Y	Y	Y	Y	N	N
14	F	57	Y	Y	N	N	N	N
15	F	44	N	Y	Y	N	N	N
16	F	42	Y	Y	Y	Y	N	N
17	M	52	N	Y	Y	Y	N	Y
18	M	54	Y	Y	Y	Y	N	Y
19	M	50	Y	Y	N	N	N	N
20	F	59	Y	Y	Y	Y	N	N
21	M	56	Y	Y	Y	Y	N	Y

Participant number	Gender (Male/Female)	Age	Muslim	Researcher	REC member	Guideline author	Islamic scholar	Informal training in Islamic sciences
22	M	48	Y	Y	Y	Y	N	N
23	M	37	Y	Y	Y	Y	N	N
24	M	50	Y	Y	Y	Y	N	N
25	F	57	Y	Y	Y	Y	N	N
26	M	38	Y	Y	Y	N	N	N
27	M	64	Y	N	Y	N	Y	N/A
28	F	43	Y	Y	N	N	N	N
29	F	51	Y	Y	Y	Y	N	N
30	M	56	Y	Y	N	Y	N	N
31	M	63	Y	Y	N	Y	N	Y
32	M	40	Y	N	Y	Y	Y	N/A
33	M	63	Y	N	N	N	Y	N/A
34	M	33	Y	Y	N	N	N	N
35	M	35	Y	Y	Y	N	N	N
36	M	33	Y	Y	N	N	N	N
37	F	30	N	Y	N	N	N	N
38a	M	52	N	Y	N	N	N	N
38b	F	49	N	Y	N	N	N	N

Table 8.2 Iran participant profile, including gender (male/female), age, researcher (Y/N), REC member (Y/N), guideline developer (Y/N), Islamic scholar (Y/N), informal training in the Islamic sciences (Y/N)

Participant number	Gender (Male/Female)	Age	Muslim	Researcher	REC member	Guideline author	Islamic scholar	Informal training in Islamic sciences
1	M	34	Y	Y	Y	Y	N	Y
2	M	70	Y	Y	Y	Y	N	Y
3	M	43	Y	Y	Y	N	N	N
4	F	41	Y	Y	Y	N	N	N
5	F	49	Y	Y	Y	N	N	N
6	M	51	Y	Y	Y	N	N	N
7	M	41	Y	Y	Y	N	N	N
8	M	45	Y	Y	Y	Y	N	Y
9	F	54	Y	Y	Y	Y	N	N
10	F	37	Y	Y	Y	N	N	Y
11	M	43	Y	Y	Y	Y	N	Y
12	F	43	Y	Y	Y	Y	N	Y
13	F	46	Y	Y	Y	Y	N	Y
14	M	47	Y	Y	Y	Y	N	N
15	M	48	Y	Y	Y	Y	N	Y
16	M	46	Y	N	Y	Y	Y	N/A
17	M	42	Y	N	Y	Y	Y	N/A

Gaining access to research participants

Ethical considerations and clearance

As the study involved direct participation involving human subjects, the following were considered appropriate ethical considerations and permissions.

I. PROCESS OF OBTAINING INFORMED CONSENT OF PARTICIPANTS

All participants were asked to read and sign a written consent form. The information sheet was sent in advance via email to allow participants the opportunity to ask questions or withdraw from the interview. Before the interview began, participants were provided with a verbal brief of the study and the opportunity to ask questions or withdraw. The interview was conducted, and an audio recording was made, only after the participant had signed the form. The participants were also informed that they could withdraw from the study at any stage.

II. CONFIDENTIALITY

Identifiable information about participants was not shared with anyone except my DPhil research supervisors. To ensure confidentiality, the names of participants are not used in this volume or other associated publications. Instead, numbers are used to identify participants. All of the documents/recordings were stored securely in locked cabinets and on password-protected computers. After completion of the research, the recordings were destroyed. I also instructed anyone present at the interview, such as translators, to keep what was said in the discussion confidential.

III. BENEFITS AND RISKS TO PARTICIPANTS

There were no benefits to participating in the study, and participation was voluntary. The interview and survey took, generally, up to one hour at a date, time and place approved by each participant to help minimize inconvenience.

IV. ETHICAL REVIEW

Ethics approval was sought from local ethics committees in Iran and Malaysia as well as the University of Oxford research ethics committee (OXTREC) (OXTREC Reference: 540–14). The ethics approval from Iran (Reference: IRAN. REC.1393.77) was completed within a month and was unproblematic, as assistance was provided by a local contact, Dr. Ehsan Shamsi, to ensure the interview guide and research method were considered appropriate for the context. A similar process was carried out in Malaysia (Reference: KPJ Date 6/9/14) with the assistance of Professor Lokman Saim. OXTREC approval was then sought and, after minor changes to the interview guide and research protocol, ethics approval was granted for the study (References: KPJUC/ECC/CPGS/11(00); IRAN.REC.1393.77). The ethical review processes were very similar for Oxford, Malaysia and Iran, and I did not encounter any "Islamic" issues when trying to obtain the ethics approval.

Two of the interviews in Iran required a translator, as the interviewees were not confident with their ability to communicate in English. The participants were comfortable with the translators appointed by the Tehran University of Medical Sciences (TUMS). One interviewee, once the interview began, realised he did not require a translator but was happy for the translator to remain within the interview. Translators were given an explanation of the research study, provided with the information sheet and asked to keep the contents of interviews confidential.

Recruitment of participants

For the Malaysia phase of the data-collection, I developed a profile of the types of participants and institutions suitable for the study. Recruitment began initially by obtaining appropriate profiles (purposive sampling) from university websites and requesting contact details of colleagues of Professor Lokman Saim. I then systematically wrote to approximately 50 potential candidates before I was due to travel to Malaysia, and I managed to secure 20 interview dates and times. Once in Malaysia I was able to employ a snowball sampling method with recommendations and contact details from interviewees, who identified colleagues they considered suitable for my study. Interview participants ranged from researchers, guideline authors, research committee members, Islamic scholars and academics involved in deliberations about research ethics in Malaysia.

Recruitment of participants in Malaysia was relatively straightforward. Many respondents expressed appreciation at having been invited into a DPhil research study. The fact that I am a medical professional and researcher may have made the initial contact via email easier than if I had been entirely external to the medical field. However, meticulous management of time and reminders to participants were necessary to ensure the interviews could be conducted on the dates and times agreed, as the study period was limited. The process, however, was successful, and there was only one instance in Malaysia where a participant did not appear for interview and was not contactable thereafter.

Interviews were conducted at locations convenient to participants, and they were commonly held at the participants' offices. When conducted in a public place, the interview setting posed the challenge of background noise, however, this rarely posed a problem, as the audio quality remained adequate for transcription. All interviews were conducted in English. Where Arabic or Malay terminology was used, the interviewee was asked, as much as possible, to translate for the benefit of the recording. There were instances where Arabic terminology was not translated by the participant because it was decided that the interruption would disturb the participants' response, and I was adequately aware of the translation and intended/common use of the terminology.

In Iran, by contrast, I was advised not to invite participants to the study until I arrived in person and was able to provide details of my study to the various institutions where participants would be recruited. Although this initially presented uncertainty in terms of recruitment and planning, once the process began, and I established a suitable rapport with administrators in the relevant institutions, recruiting participants of different levels of seniority and experience was relatively unproblematic.

In both countries, it was a challenge to recruit formally recognised Islamic scholars. Although I systematically contacted RECs and relevant institutions (e.g., Islamic studies departments, seminaries, *fatwah* councils) in both countries, I either received no replies or was informed (either by email or phone call) that the scholars were busy and/or unavailable during my visit. I did manage, however, to interview three Islamic scholars in Malaysia and two in Iran. These interviews were very rich, and they were supplemented by the views of researchers and REC members, who though not formally recognised as scholars, were informally trained in the Islamic sciences and had published and taught extensively on the subject.

Research instruments

For in-depth interviews with participants, an open-ended, thematic interview guide was developed (see the Appendix) to ensure that the same themes were covered in each of the five interview tiers. The guide provided flexibility, however, to ensure that questioning could occur freely while allowing the interviewer to choose questions appropriate to the context and enabling suitable probing of topics and issues that were pertinent and that arose within the interview.

Table 8.3 illustrates the rationale of the topic guide, combining themes from the literature and guideline review and open-ended questions to yield novel ethical issues. As can be seen, the interviews generally began with more of an open discussion and, depending on the participants' responses and the background from the literature and guidelines, more specific questions were asked as necessary to probe further according to the participants' responses. Most participants were asked about their views on topics found in the literature and guideline review, and if they had consulted an Islamic scholar/*fatwah* (legal edict) during their consideration of ethical issues encountered within the research setting.

Additionally, a survey was completed to collect socio-demographic information from all of the participants (see Tables 8.1 and 8.2 above). For the Muslim participants, it included additional questions about their religiosity (Huber & Huber, 2012), and references to the Islamic tradition both within the personal and practical sphere were incorporated into the questionnaire. As explained above, the latter was implemented only in Malaysia.

Qualitative data collection methods

Having developed the interview guide, I tested its coherence and the timing of the questioning by conducting three preliminary interviews (Silverman, 2013, p. 124).

Table 8.3 Rationale for the semi-structured interview guide showing themes that were derived from the literature and guidelines

	Introduction and a brief description of what the research is about	What is your experience of clinical research?
Open questions	Part A:	What kinds of difficult decisions do you face in your work? Can you tell me more about these?
		What resources do you have/use to navigate through such questions? Are there guidelines/laws?
More specific questions relating to Islam's role in personal decision-making	Part B: Islam as personal faith	Does your faith (or the faith of others) influence what you consider to be an ethical/moral problem?
		Do you think faith is important in defining what an ethical/ problem is in the context of research?
		Is it necessary to consider faith when ensuring that research is conducted ethically? Why? Why not?
More specific questions related to the institutional aspects of Islam	Part C: Institutional aspects of Islam and their authority	What role, if any, does Islam play in the national law and national prioritisation for health and health research?
		Does Islamic ethics impact research priorities, research guideline production and research conduct? If so, how? If not, why not?
		Have you ever referred to an Islamic scholar when faced with a question in biomedical research?
		Have you ever referred to a *fatwah* or *fatwah* council when faced with a question in biomedical research?

More specific questions related to topics encountered in the literature and guidelines, including:		
(i) HIV research	Part D: Case studies of particular issues in research ethics	In the literature, and during my discussion with others, it has been mentioned that there are certain types of research that cannot be done in Muslim contexts, e.g., looking at the efficacy of HIV prevention programmes using contraception, as this promotes promiscuity in the society. Have you ever come across this or other such issues, and could you tell me more about these?
(ii) Enrolling women into research studies		Have you ever encountered any challenges when trying to conduct research studies involving female participants? Can you describe some of these challenges?
		Are there any particular studies that would be difficult to carry out that involve women?
		Some literature suggests that before women are enrolled into a study, the researcher or participant should seek permission from her husband or male guardian? What are your views on this? Can you explain to me why?

These were invaluable in allowing me to assess and reflect on the experience of interviewing and highlighting the need to keep the topic guide flexible to allow the discussion to remain focused on the participants' experiences, rather than being simply led by the pre-existing topics.

In Malaysia, I began by conducting three interviews, which I then discussed with my supervisors to make necessary amendments to the guide. The amendments reflected the experience of the Malaysian researchers in comparison to the preliminary interviewees, where specific topics were reserved for the end of the discussion if the participant required more prompting for the exploration of particular themes.

In Iran, a similar method was employed to primarily assess whether the same interview guide was suitable to explore the ethical questions encountered by participants and their views on how these were addressed. Within the first three interviews, it became clear that the guide was sufficient, and the method employed in Malaysia was suitable in Iran, with relevant contextual adaptations.

The order in which themes were discussed varied between each interview in order to allow respondents flexibility and ensure that the questioning and probing were reflective of the responses. This was considered important, as flexibility enables the capturing of respondents' own ideas and reflections (Denscombe, 2014, pp. 184–204), allows participants to feel they have ownership of their responses and assures them that their contributions are valued and considered pertinent to the research question. This method assisted in the building of rapport with the participants. Even when respondents were initially hesitant, when they were able to talk freely, without being interrupted or directed, they were able to express in detail ethical questions from their own experiences.

Data analysis methods

Semi-structured interviews

Semi-structured interviews were audio recorded and transcribed. Using data from notes taken at the interviews and transcriptions of the audio recordings, a framework analysis approach was employed (Green et al., 2013, pp. 209–17; Pope et al., 2000). The method I used reflects the framework analysis requirements described first by Ritchie and Lewis (2003), who suggest that the framework should ensure the investigator:

1   Remains grounded in the data
2   Permits captured synthesis – this is reflected in the charting process where verbatim text is reduced from its raw form
3   Facilitates and displays ordering – again, this is reflected in the charting process
4   Permits within and between case searches – the charting process allows for searching and comparisons to be made within and between data sets (p. 56).

Such a method ensures that the data analysis process is systematic, comprehensive and flexible to enable new ideas to be generated. It also enables refinements and ensures transparency to others. Ritchie and Lewis's method of analysis is one that involves an "analytical hierarchy", which begins with familiarisation of the data or data management, followed by the generation of descriptive accounts and, finally, abstraction through the development of explanatory accounts (Ritchie & Lewis, 2003, p. 56). The following describes how I carried out these steps of analysis:

1   Familiarisation with the data – this first step was employed to ensure, as primary investigator, I remained close to the data. This involved immersion in the data, with repeated reading of field notes, summaries and transcripts, in order to list key ideas, recurrent themes and patterns. I did not code at this stage. Instead, I summarised the key points participants made via a summary sheet for each interview. Each of the transcripts was discussed with my supervisors during the interview period to enable me to develop an initial systematic reflection of the data.

2   Generating themes – a coding scheme was developed by identifying all the key issues, concepts and themes. This was carried out by drawing on a priori issues and questions derived from the aims and objectives of the study, the literature and guideline review, as well as emergent issues raised by the participants. The coding framework was discussed with and reviewed by my supervisors. A priori issues included those from the literature, such as research, retention and sharing of genetic material, and the use of illicit substances, e.g., porcine products in vaccines. These codes were useful for generating themes about how Islam influences biomedical research ethics. During the coding process, inductive codes – those emerging from the data – were added to the coding framework if they described a new theme or expanded upon a predetermined code.

3   Indexing – the themes in the data were used as labels for codes, which were then applied to the whole data set. This was done systematically to ensure all the data were accurately coded using NVIVO version 10. The process of generating themes and indexing continued until the point of data saturation. Data saturation was assessed at the point where "no new information or themes" (Guest et al., 2006) were observed in the data. After this point, only indexing continued until all of the data had been coded. Data saturation occurred by interview 35 in Malaysia, however, I conducted an additional three interviews in order to ensure that no new themes were generated. In Iran, data saturation occurred by interview 15, however, I conducted an additional three interviews to ensure data saturation had been reached.

4   Charting (descriptive accounts) – after coding the data according to the identified themes, the data was then charted to assist in the generation of descriptive accounts where verbatim text was reduced from its raw form. This involved a rearrangement of the data according to thematic content through comparison of data within and between interviews. Once judged to be comprehensive, each main theme was charted by completing a matrix, where each

interview had its own row, and columns represented the subtopics. These charts contain summaries of data that can be referenced back to the original transcript. This enabled a presentation of the range and diversity of views. Key quotes were recorded, and certain themes were listed in the participants' own language. This was then followed by a refinement of categories to address overlap and to develop typologies, which assisted in the collation of the related themes and helped to divide and unite the participants' views. A schematic of the coding framework is illustrated in Table 8.4.

5   Mapping and interpretation (developing exploratory accounts) – the charts were then used to examine the data for patterns and connections. This stage was influenced by the original aims and objectives of the study as well as emergent issues from the data. Patterns in the data were identified to derive explanations of participants' experiences in the two case study sites by comparing the sites and the views within each site. An account was developed to explain reasons behind the differences and similarities seen in the two case study sites, and how such a comparison may impact the understanding of Islam's influence on ethical decision-making in such contexts. For example, recurrent themes were identified, and the reasons for these were explored. Explanations and reasoning given by participants were also studied in order to distinguish these from my own analysis as the investigator. This distinction is further explored below in the section on ethical analysis.

Managing as a DPhil student undertaking single coder analysis

As I was undertaking the organisation of the study as well as the interviews independently, I had to deal with the issue of ensuring reflexivity and objectivity. I kept detailed field notes in Malaysia and Iran, in between the fieldwork placements and for a few weeks after data collection was complete. This was to enable me to reflect on my interaction with the participants, my impressions of the research sites and my role as a researcher. I had lengthy and regular discussions with my supervisors, who read all of the interview transcripts and were involved in commenting on and encouraging me to critically reflect upon the development of the coding framework. We discussed and tried the coding framework for each of the transcripts and carefully considered the themes as well as the issue of data saturation. I also discussed and reflected upon my role as a Muslim female researcher with my supervisors in order to consider how my own experience and values may have transformed into the data analysis (Hobbs & Wright, 2006). A more detailed account of my reflections about my identity as a researcher as well as associated limitations is presented in subsequent sections in this chapter.

Questionnaire

A religiosity questionnaire was adapted from the work of Huber and Huber (2012) to assist in the selection of participants with a range of ritualistic religious observance and beliefs. As explained above, the questionnaire was only employed in Malaysia, as it was not considered contextually appropriate in Iran.

Table 8.4 A schematic of the coding framework

Codes	Themes/descriptive accounts	Exploratory accounts	Main themes or aspects
Living in a Muslim country, we need to consider everything from the perspective of Islamic law The REC ensures that research does not contravene Islamic law	1. Islamic ethico-legal issues emerging from personal experience 2. Islamic ethico-legal issues emerging from RECs	The role of Islam and its normative sources in how ethical issues are identified and raised by RECs and researchers	The institutional forms of Islam in bio-medical research ethics
When senior Muslim members of RECs raise a concern about an issue being against Islamic law, we need to consult a religious scholar or the *fatwah* council We need scholars to convince the public about health interventions When we were writing the guidelines we needed to consult scholars to ensure the guidelines were in keeping with Islamic law and would be acceptable to the wider public It is difficult for Islamic scholars to know the complexities of biomedicine and for physicians to know the requirements of Islamic ethics and law. Some have to train in both fields to act as a bridge between the two specialties Some researchers have knowledge of the Islamic sciences and need to act as expert witnesses at the *fatwah* council when the latter were deciding on the permissibility of needle exchange programmes	3. Role of Islamic scholars in RECs and national committees 4. Community engagement role of scholars 5. Role of scholars in the authorship of guidelines 6. Role of bridge scholars 7. Role of contextual scholars	The role of Islam and its normative sources in how ethical issues are addressed once identified by RECs and researchers	
We need to get a *fatwah* so the public know that the research is permissible according to Islamic law	8. Role of the *Shariah* and *fatwah* council 9. Motivations for seeking *fatawah*		

Islamic responses to the ethical issues of HIV/AIDS	the global health challenge of curbing the spread of HIV/AIDS poses questions for the institutional forms of Islam	about the investigation of illicit practices	the prevalence of drug use or the efficacy of needle exchange programmes
			We must try and curb HIV/AIDS but also uphold Islamic law
		11. Variations in views about how to research and address the HIV/AIDS epidemic	HIV/AIDS is prevalent in this country and we must do what we can to address this problem
	Practical deliberation using *ijtihad* to derive *fatawah* as a mechanism of addressing ethical issues of HIV/AIDS	12. Employing the principle of public good (*Maslaha*) to address the ethical issues of HIV/AIDS in Iran	Islamic law includes the principle of *Maslaha*, or public good, which scholars use to derive permission for needle exchange programmes
		13. The higher objectives of Islamic law as a means of addressing the ethical issues of HIV/AIDS in Malaysia	The higher objectives of the *Shariah* include the necessity to preserve life, which allows the implementation of needle exchange programmes
	Researching and addressing HIV/AIDS in sex workers and the LGBT community – a gap in the mechanism of Islamic ethico-legal analysis in Malaysia and Iran	14. Barriers to researching and meeting the health needs of MSMs	Homosexuality is illegal in Islam, so we cannot research HIV/AIDS amongst men who have sex with men (MSMs)
		15. Barriers to researching and meeting the health needs of sex workers	Extra marital relations are illegal in Islam, so we cannot research the prevalence of practices of sex workers
Women's participation in biomedical research	The role and status of women and the appropriation of Islamic normative texts in biomedical research ethics	16. Autonomy and consent of Muslim female research participants	If I am enrolling a female participant into a trial and her husband disagrees, then I will not pursue the enrolment
		17. Understanding autonomy and the concepts of *Wilayah, Qiwamah, Ta'ah and Nushuz*	Even if her husband disagrees, it is the woman's right to decide whether or not she wants to enrol
			The *Qur'an* mentions that men need to protect their women, so if the husband prefers her not to enrol, then she will not be enrolled into the trial
			A woman cannot leave the house without her husband's permission
	Challenges relating to women's health and wellbeing	18. Intimate and domestic partner violence	Women think that they need to be obedient to their husbands, and the *Qur'an* allows husbands to hit their wives
		19. Women's sexual health and sexual experience	Women believe they must keep what happens in their homes and their bedrooms private

I cannot do research on issues like sex work, as that is illegal in Islam	20. Conscientious objection and beliefs about legal and moral accountability in HIV/AIDS research	Practical deliberations involving personal and professional values – HIV/AIDS
I cannot do something that is illegal in Islam, as I will then have to account for it in the "hereafter"	21. Advocacy role of biomedical researchers in the process of *ijtihad* and deriving *fatawah* for addressing HIV/AIDS	
My responsibility as a doctor and health researcher is my main priority, so I have to speak to Islamic scholars to try and convince them that implementing a needle exchange programme is essential for curbing HIV/AIDS		
When I do research on intimate and domestic partner violence, I am not sure about how to speak to the women about obedience	22. Moral consciousness and moral anxiety when researching and meeting the health needs of women	Practical deliberations involving personal and professional values – women's health and enrolment into research
Islam does not condone violence against women, but how do I tell women about issues that relate to their beliefs?		

Practical deliberations involving personal and professional values

Direct observation

Non-participant observation was used to capture information about the different contexts, organisations and interactions.

Ethical analysis

It is important to consider, in addition to the above data analysis, what the role of an ethical analysis was in this project. Ethical analysis here does not mean doing normative ethics. It means developing, on the basis of the data, a rich empirical account of the roles that ethics plays in the lives and thinking of the participants, such as what poses an ethical problem for them, and how they go about addressing it? Although participants may outline what they consider to be ethical problems or characterise the sorts of ethical questions they encounter and how they address these, it was also the aim of this study to reflect on the intellectual deliberations of participants. This was to allow an abstract consideration of the ethical challenges that may be emergent within the study sites that can be reflected on. The latter was done based on my understanding and reading of abstract ethical principles. Such an analysis was conducted to enable a cross-reference between the empirical data offered by the research participants and the relevant normative ethical debates. These includes some of the topics discussed in Chapter 1, including universalism and relativism, the ethical relevance of distinguishing between religion and culture and role of moral perceptions and particularity.

This process of analysis allowed me to reflect on whether and how Islam influences biomedical research ethics, and whether there are distinct ethical concerns and methods of deliberation that arise as a result of considering Islam and its institutional forms. It also enabled me to assess how Islam and its institutional forms are appropriated for ethical deliberations within the biomedical research context by researchers, REC members, guideline developers and Islamic scholars.

The ethical analysis of this study had two aims, which included:

1   Providing an analysis of the participants' understanding of normative ethical principles, with a reflection on their moral perspectives and values about what they consider to be ethical questions/problems, and how these compare with the existing bioethical literature.
2   To reflect on the accounts offered by participants, in terms of their questions and modes of tackling such issues, to develop my own account of what ethical challenges exist and/or arise within these contexts.

Ethical reflections on the methods of this study

This section briefly outlines some of the ethical considerations and dilemmas that arose for me as I planned, conducted and evaluated my fieldwork experience. As the fieldwork involved an exploration of the influence of the institutional aspects of Islam as well as personal faith in the understanding of ethical issues in research, throughout the process I had to reflect on the probable ethical challenges I would encounter, and how to best prepare for these. In both Malaysia and Iran, the history of Islam, its political and social role as well as its personal commitment and expression are complex and sensitive. I tried to speak to other DPhil students who had worked in the same or similar contexts, as well as other researchers who had worked in Malaysia and Iran, to discuss how best to prepare for my fieldwork. This planning process was invaluable in ensuring I had the necessary time and resources to organise adequately for both field visits.

Some of the initial ethical concerns I considered included the ability of participants to freely agree to participate in such a study, and if they did consent, then the ability to ensure that they were able to express their views unreservedly. As one of the objectives of the study was to better understand the role of personal faith in the context of specific ethical issues, I was keen to ensure that participants were comfortable sharing their views and experiences. The latter required participants being sufficiently reassured that their contributions would remain confidential and anonymous, and my communicating that if they wished to withdraw, they would be able to at any point. I spent time ensuring that the information sheet and consent form detailed such arrangements, and I also informed the participants of these before each interview.

During a few interviews in Malaysia, participants expressed views that challenged existing institutional, political and/or religious authorities. They did not retract such views, however, they emphasised that they would like to remain anonymous and would not like their institutions mentioned. I explained again that the data would remain confidential and that their views would only be identified by number, and that their institution would not be listed next to their views, if quoted in publications such as this volume. All of the participants were satisfied with this explanation and were very happy to express their views freely.

In Iran, there was one instance where a participant asked me to stop recording the interview but was happy to speak to me about her experiences of Islamic scholarly involvement in RECs and guideline development. The participant said she was happy for me to take notes of her views and to use these within my analysis, but not to have an audio recording or to quote her verbatim. She explained that the role of Islamic scholars in Iran is politically sensitive, and she did not want her views to be traced back to her or her institution. Given her concerns, during the interview I stopped both recorders at the point of her request and took notes of her views and experiences. When she had finished discussing the role of scholars and was happy for me to do so, I restarted the recording. Although in other interviews in Iran participants expressed similar views and concerns about the role of Islamic scholars, all of the respondents were comfortable with the audio recording.

Having local contacts check my invitation letters, consent forms and information sheets, as well as mentioning them on the documentation, was critical in ensuring that when participants were approached, they were aware that the study had been locally approved and vetted. And if there had been instances where participants were unhappy with the research encounter, then they could consult the local contact, as well as my supervisors and myself. Such a need did not arise during the fieldwork; however, it was important to make such arrangements.

In Iran, the question of exploring people's expressed religiosity through the questionnaire was not initially considered to be a problem at the time I planned the field visit. However, upon my arrival I spoke to two participants, and they explained that such a questionnaire would likely cause anxiety and hamper the main source of data collection, the interviews. As the religiosity questionnaire was not central to the data collection, it was important to withdraw it as a data collection tool to remain respectful of local concerns around the political implications of expressed religiosity as well as to take into account the advice that I had received.

In one of the interviews in Malaysia, the participant became upset and emotional when expressing the challenges she had experienced when trying to conduct research on women's sexual health and sexual experiences. I stopped recording the interview and asked her whether she would like to have a break or to continue the interview at a later date. She reassured me that she would like to carry on and, in fact, stated that she found the interview process helpful, as she had been unable to discuss her anxieties and experiences with her colleagues. As the interview continued, the participant became more relaxed and was able to articulate her views and the barriers she had encountered when researching women's sexual health in Malaysia. It was difficult to simply consider this encounter as a researcher-participant relationship. At the end of the interview, the participant asked me about my experiences as a Muslim female researcher myself. I was able to share with her some of my personal experiences of my DPhil research, and I offered to see her again informally. The participant reassured me that the interview was not a negative experience for her; rather, she said that it was reassuring to speak to someone she could relate to. This interview was the only encounter I had during my fieldwork where the participant was visibly affected during the meeting. She explained that her emotional response was not due to any specific question or probing; rather, it was the first time she had been able to articulate her own views and experiences, which caused her to be upset. I was mindful of this meeting throughout my subsequent interviews and ensured that I was able to give time to participants and to be attentive towards non-verbal cues that may have indicated their anxiety.

In both countries, I was concerned that my being visibly Muslim may have unduly affected participants' responses. However, I found that in both Malaysia and Iran participants were keen and able to share their concerns and anxieties about the role of Islamic scholars, the political influence of Islamisation and Muslim identity within their context. In both countries participants expressed when they did not consider their faith as being necessary or if they thought the influence of Islam and its formative elements were unhelpful in the context of biomedical research.

Reflections on my identity as a researcher

Given the above ethical reflections and the aforementioned recognition of my role as a researcher, I will briefly discuss the considerations that were made regarding my pre-existing values and experiences, how these were discussed at length with my supervisors and how they were catalogued through detailed field notes to ensure that I was able to be reflective and retain a professional distance from the data and interviewee accounts in order to enable objective analysis. It is recognised that in qualitative studies, the researcher's "identity, values, and beliefs" (Denscombe, 2014, p. 89) cannot be excluded as an influence in the process of data gathering and analysis as well the process of interpretation and abstraction. In acknowledgement of this, a number of strategies were developed and implemented for ensuring critical reflexivity or awareness about pre-existing experiences, interests and motivations of the qualitative researcher in relation to the research aims and objectives as well as the processes of data collection, analysis and interpretation (Bourdieu, 2004). The following is an account of my personal identity, beliefs and experiences that may have been pertinent to this research, which may enable the reader to better understand my role in the research process.

Being medically trained and having lived and worked in sub-Saharan Africa, I was familiar with global health challenges, such as HIV/AIDS, and barriers to accessing healthcare resources in resource-poor settings and by those from marginalised groups. Prior to the DPhil, I had completed an MSc in Global Health Sciences and had carried out a qualitative research project on factors influencing participation in research in Kenya. This background equipped me to synthesise the literature relating to biomedical research ethics and enabled me to undertake the ethical analysis described above. I am also a practising Muslim who has been studying the Islamic sciences for over ten years. A familiarity with the primary texts and the derived sciences was incredibly useful in facilitating probing during interviews with Islamic scholars and other participants who employed verses from the *Qur'an* or traditions of the Prophet to explain their ethico-legal deliberations. This background was also useful for the literature and guideline review, as many of the references found cited primary and/or secondary Islamic sources. Part of the analysis was to evaluate the role of the Islamic sciences in the literature and guidelines, and as I was familiar with the Islamic sciences, I was able to confidently navigate through such references.

Despite such advantages, I had to be aware of the potential drawbacks and impact of my identity as a researcher on the literature and guideline review, the interview process as well as the data analysis. With regards to the literature and guideline review, I ensured that I designed the search strategy in consultation with an experienced information scientist and discussed the findings and analysis at length with my supervisors. During the fieldwork, I was very open with participants about my having been educated in the UK and having an interest in biomedical research ethics. As a visibly Muslim woman, participants were able to immediately recognise my commitment to my faith. Being transparent about these main aspects of myself was very helpful in ensuring that participants were able to know and ask about my motivations for conducting this study. Many did ask, either at the start or the end of the interview, about why a medically trained professional would conduct social science research. I explained that I was interested in how people make decisions and, while much had been written about clinical decision-making, there is very little scholarship about researchers' ethical deliberations. Many of the participants welcomed my explanations, and this helped build a rapport between myself, the participants and the wider biomedical research community that I interacted with whilst I was in the two case study sites.

Being Muslim also meant that participants commonly asked me what I thought about the issues they encountered. I carefully informed them that the purpose of the interview was to collect their impressions and accounts. I did offer some personal reflections at the end of the interview, however, particularly in the case of the Muslim female researcher described above who had experienced a challenging professional environment. Such discussions consisted of me sharing my experience of living and working in the UK, particularly in Oxford, as all of the participants were familiar with the university. I was very careful in ensuring that I only had such discussions after the interview, as I wanted to reassure the participants that the interview process was to capture their views, and I wanted to prevent any bias in their responses through my own interjections.

Given my background, I also ensured that each interview began with open questions where participants were able to discuss the challenges and questions they themselves had encountered. I then probed why they considered these to be challenges and how they went about addressing them. I also then carefully asked what resources they had to deal with such issues, and whether there were gaps in them being able to adequately address the issues they faced. It was through participant-led discussions that the issues of HIV/AIDS and the role of women in research became apparent as recurring themes. These two themes were also prevalent in the literature. When I discussed the transcripts from both Malaysia and Iran with my supervisors, we all agreed that these two themes were prominent in participants' accounts of the challenges that they face in the biomedical research context.

I also reflected on how speaking to male Islamic scholars about ethical issues seemed daunting to me at first. However, I found that all of the scholars – in fact, all of the participants – were incredibly respectful of the research I was trying to conduct, and they were very forthcoming in sharing their views. Being female, I had to be mindful of the themes and emphasis throughout the interview process. Although one of the predominant themes within the interviews was about women's health research, most of the participants offered their accounts of this topic independently. As encountered in the literature, the role and status of women is disputed in Islam and throughout the Muslim world. All of the participants were familiar with these debates within their own contexts, and they were keen to share their perspectives on women's health research.

I did spend time deliberating about how best to capture rich accounts whilst giving participants enough information about the study itself so that they could offer views and experiences relevant to the research question. I tried to send the information sheet well in advance of the interview. Although I did probe participants about what they considered to be ethical problems and why, I was very careful to not offer my own opinions or to probe towards a consensus. While I was familiar with the challenges of HIV/AIDS in sub-Saharan Africa and there was a risk that my background could draw me to topics that I was familiar with, I reflected with my supervisors on this possibility throughout the process of analysis, and I am confident from the interview data that they provide convincing evidence that the ethical issues surrounding HIV/AIDS have been very topical in Malaysia and Iran. Again, participants commonly used the epidemic as a case study to explain ethical issues they had encountered and how they addressed them.

To ensure transparency, I was keen to share my findings with participants, and I presented a preliminary analysis of my data in both Malaysia and Iran. The presentations were well received by the participants who were able to attend. I did not send transcripts to participants for review because, when asked, they stated that it would take up too much of their time. However, I shared the final DPhil findings with all of the participants who were keen to receive them.

I did ensure that each of the transcripts was carefully discussed with my supervisors, the themes and codes reviewed repeatedly and the four key themes that were identified were the most predominant in the participant accounts and encountered in the literature review. Despite such methodological considerations, it is important to reflect on the potential biases that may have resulted from my identity as a researcher. A more detailed discussion of these limitations is presented in this chapter.

Data analysis and the process of developing the four main themes of the study

Having analysed the literature and guidelines, completed the interviews and studied the transcripts using a framework analysis, I identified four key themes that helped me organise the insights emerging from the data. Although the data could have been presented in multiple ways, and I drafted several versions of the data tables and the data chapters, the themes outlined below ultimately functioned best as organising concepts for the data I gathered from the participants I interviewed. The four themes are as follows:

a   Authority in Islam and its influence on biomedical research – relating to the role of Islamic scholars, texts and legal edicts.
b   HIV, sexuality and sexual health research – relating to ethical concerns about issues considered illegal in Islam as well as professional concerns/obligations and deliberations about benefits and harms.
c   Women's participation in research – relating to concerns about autonomy, the role of the family as well as the role and status of women in Islam.
d   Personal faith – relating to participants' personal deliberations about biomedical research priorities and how these are balanced against their personal understanding of religious, cultural and other obligations/sources of moral reasoning.

Whilst these themes emerged as being important from my analysis of participant accounts, they also provided a framework through which the data and discussion from this study could be related back to the broader bioethical discussions around universal versus relative ethical principles, the balancing of professional and personal ethical priorities that were introduced in Chapter 1 and the guideline review presented in Chapter 2.

In addition to the four mentioned themes, there was a large list of nodes and sub-nodes during the coding process, which represented the numerous topics that were encountered in the interviews. These were largely organised into topics/themes/ethical issues that were "Islamic" or "non-Islamic". The rationale for this categorisation was that it reflected participants' labelling of a topic or ethical issue as "Islamic". Alternatively, when I analysed their deliberations, if I found that the reasoning relied overtly on primary and/or secondary normative sources of Islam, for example, where they included quotations of *Qur'an* verses or specific *Hadith*, such topics/themes/ethical issues were labelled as "Islamic". Participants also mentioned topics as "non-Islamic", i.e., as being (in their opinion) independent of their consideration of Islam, e.g., issues that depended on professional, national or global biomedical research guidelines/priorities. For example, many participants referred to the principle of justice, as encountered specifically in the work of Beauchamp and Childress (2001). They argued that it played a role in their ethical decision-making, and the understanding and application of this principle did not rely on any "Islamic" sources per se.

A number of non-Islamic and Islamic ethico-legal issues emerged from the analysis of the data:

Non-Islamic ethical issues, i.e., those identified by participants as being (for them) considerations independent of Islam:

- RECs and their role
- Consent
- Scientific validity/method
- Benefits and harms
- Justice
- Duty of care/professional obligation
- Concerns about current system/infrastructure

Ethical issues identified by participants as "Islamic":

- Matters considered illegal according to Islamic law, e.g., use or consumption of alcohol, extramarital sex, homosexuality
- Theological matters, e.g., when does life begin and end?
- Scientific study/method – concerns driven by personal beliefs of researcher/REC member, e.g., intentions for doing research
- Professional concerns/obligations – concerns driven by personal beliefs of researcher/REC member, e.g., concerns about studying illicit behaviours, such as IV drug use
- Family – relating to autonomy, collective decision-making and participation of women in research
- Benefits and harms – concerns driven by personal beliefs of participants/research community/researchers/REC members, e.g., concerns about a research study condoning illicit practices
- Religious obligations, e.g., issues relating to prayer and fasting

- Role of authority – involvement of and concerns about the role of Islamic scholars and their edicts

The data analysis showed that many of the ethical issues encountered by the research participants in this study are common to researchers elsewhere (Emanuel et al., 2000). However, what emerged from the data was that Islam, its institutional forms and its associated practices were particularly important when participants were deliberating ethical issues in research that had a bearing on Islam's legal or theological instructions or that had less openly discussed traditional/cultural roots.

Other themes and topics were considered important; however, as the presentation of the data required me to focus on and present a limited amount of information, I had to undertake a process of repeatedly analysing the data and reflecting on the richness, depth and breadth of participant accounts (Chenail, 1995). For a word-limited publication (Chenail, 1995), therefore, I had to rely on the following parameters to select the four key themes around which the data chapters were organised:

1   Do they answer the study question (Sandelowski, 1998)?
2   Do participants consider them important?
3   Do they enable presentation of what is prevalent in the data as well as rich accounts and explanations (Chenail, 1995; Sandelowski, 1998)?
4   Do they cohere with findings from the literature and guideline review (Chenail, 1995)?
5   Do they provide a framework through which the data and discussion from this study could be related back to the broader bioethical discussions around universal versus relative ethical principles and the balancing of professional and personal ethical priorities, which were introduced in Chapter 1 (Chenail, 1995)?

The four themes were chosen as they aligned with these five parameters and, most critically, were emphasised by participants as being particularly important in their work and deliberations around biomedical research ethics.

Presenting the data – how quotes were chosen

For evidencing the findings and illustrating perspectives of participants (Sandelowski, 1994), quotes were carefully chosen for presentation in the data chapters. However, in keeping with the "aesthetics and ethics" (Sandelowski, 1994) of qualitative research reporting, as some of the participant explanations were lengthy, quotes had to be selected that were relevant for each section. Sometimes they were edited for readability, grammar and brevity. I was careful, however, to select and edit quotes to retain the overall message of each transcript from which they were extracted. I kept detailed memos during the coding process to assist the selection of appropriate quotes.

Limitations of this research

Limitations of the guideline review

As the guideline review was limited to online sources identified through Google searches, email contact or the OHRP database, the data gathered was inevitably limited to some extent. Guidelines and policies not available online were excluded, i.e., those only available in print. As these were not accessed, this limited the number of guidelines that were available for review. Another limitation was that, although all of the ministries were contacted, very few replied with details about whether and what guidelines they use. Also, it is important to point out here that countries that do not have bespoke guidelines may simply implement international guidelines, such as CIOMS. Without verification, it is not possible to conclude whether such countries have/use research ethics guidelines.

Another limitation was that non-English guidelines were excluded. This limited the number of guidelines I was able to review. Further work needs to be conducted to more comprehensively include non-English guidelines as well as guidelines that are only available in print. Another limitation of the guideline review was that the study was limited to guidelines within the OIC. A significant number of Muslims live in North America, Europe and other countries that are not members of the OIC. Future work may shed light on research ethics guidelines outside of the OIC and whether they incorporate "Islamic" values.

Limitations of the empirical study

There are numerous limitations in relation to the methods employed for the empirical study. I defined the "Muslim world" and restricted the sampling of potential sites to countries within the OIC. The OIC is comprised of countries that have a substantial Muslim population. Excluding the significant minorities of Muslims that live within Europe, North America and India from the sampling frame limits the generalizability of the findings of this research and points to a need for research within these other contexts. The study was also limited to two case study sites. Further research is needed in other OIC countries to investigate the role of Islam on biomedical research ethics and assess the extent to which the findings in this study are transferable to different sites.

Sampling and recruitment were also limited to researchers, REC members, research guideline developers and Islamic scholars. Other stakeholders involved in deliberations relating to biomedical research ethics whose views were not included in this study may include, for example, funders and research participants. Again, their absence limits the generalizability of the study's findings, and future research may provide a means of addressing this gap.

Also, there are limitations of the study relating to the scope and depth of the data collection method. I chose a combination of Malaysia and Iran and, within these sites, a broad range of institutions and organisations to both enable an in-depth study of the individual case study sites and capture the breadth of views and experiences. Two countries and 50+ participants cannot be representative of the two case study sites, Islam or the views and challenges that are prevalent in other Islamic contexts. Also, some of the ethico-legal issues encountered by participants in the case study sites may be context specific. This limits the ability to apply the findings to other populations or to Islam as a whole.

Although a widely used religiosity questionnaire (Huber & Huber, 2012) was employed during the data collection phase in Malaysia, there were limitations to its use in Iran due to local concerns around expressed religiosity. The quantitative religiosity survey developed by Huber and Huber (2012) was used to optimise recruitment of Muslim participants in Malaysia by attempting to capture the views of a mixture of religious and non-religious participants. The authors kindly provided a version of the questionnaire that they specifically use for Muslim participants in Islamic/Muslim contexts. However, a recent study argues that religiosity questionnaires like that developed by Huber and Huber (2012) have limited application for Muslim contexts as they "simply translated indicators measuring Christian religiosity into Islamic terminology" (El-Menouar & Stiftung, 2014, p. 53). Although participants in Malaysia did not express discomfort or problems when filing out the questionnaire, and the results were not used as a means of excluding participants, the experience in Iran illustrates that such questionnaires may not be appropriate in every context. El-Menouar & Stiftung's (2014) work also indicates that the questionnaire they developed specifically accommodates "the characteristics of Islamic piety" (p. 53), which may be considered more suitable for other contexts. Although the scope of this research was not to assess the appropriateness of the religiosity questionnaire devised by Huber and Huber (2012), future studies may provide more insights into religiosity questionnaires within the context of biomedical research ethics.

Another very important limitation to consider is in relation to my role as a researcher. As discussed above, I carry my own experiences, values and interpretative capability, and a combination of these were present throughout the study period. Although I kept detailed field notes in order to document my reflections and discussed them at length with my supervisors, it is important to consider how my own understandings and interests may have influenced the overall data collection, analysis and conclusions of this research. The four main themes identified were heavily dependent on the literature, guidelines and participant accounts. However, other themes that were found during the interviews, such as research fraud or the role of religious obligations, may not have been given the full weight they could have been given during the data collection phase and analysis. Although I tried to remain constantly reflexive in order to maximize objectivity, this limitation cannot be overlooked.

Another limitation is that, although interviews were used as the method of data collection, and it was explained why such an approach was appropriate for this study, there are other types of data that would have added to the richness of and further analysis within such a study. For example, during the field visits REC members and chairs mentioned that, within REC meetings in Malaysia and Iran, deliberations on ethical issues are recorded in minutes or detailed within transcripts. Although I sought permission to access these files whilst visiting the different institutions, I was informed that the data were confidential. If I did want to gain access, then it would require careful planning and the seeking of appropriate permissions. In hindsight, it would have been invaluable to have access to this data. Future research studies may want to incorporate a process for gaining access to such data alongside or within the ethics approval process for studies.

An additional limitation is that, in order to address the concern that people's understanding of what is considered an ethical issue varies, the words "challenge" or "difficult issues/decisions" were used to raise the question of whether participants had encountered ethical issues in their work. The approach was used to help broaden the type and scope of responses that participants could offer, particularly if the participants did not consider a particular issue or question or challenge as being ethically relevant. However, this broad-brush approach meant that participants sometimes raised concerns that were not ethically relevant and that were wider concerns about research, such as securing funding. Although such concerns were invaluable in providing a more detailed contextual picture of participants' responses, occasionally such responses took time away from the more ethically problematic issues or led me to ask about whether they had encountered the topics in the interview guide (female consent, HIV/AIDS, use of *fatawah* – see the Appendix), which may have prevented the collection of wider ethical issues faced by participants.

Another limitation, which relates to the above, is that participants were not sent the topic guide before the interviews. The information sheet provided a broad outline of the research objectives and methods; however, the precise questions and topics were not included. This was to enable me to document participants' own descriptions, analyses of events and explanations of the practical deliberations they undertake in an organic, unrehearsed manner. It was to also encourage participants to offer a more diverse range of issues than was included in the interview guide. I was concerned that sending the topic guide in advance may have led to bias in the data collection. However, this approach meant that, given the time constraints of the interviews, it took some participants a long time to connect the questions they encountered with the underlying ethical problems and, at times, connection was not possible, therefore I had to infer what the underlying ethical problem may have been. Although many of the participants were REC members and had training in research ethics, very few were ethicists. Some found it difficult to articulate an account of the ethical problems they encountered and how they addressed them. However, in such cases, topics from the interview guide were used to ascertain firstly whether the participants had faced a similar problem and, if so, to provide them with the opportunity to elaborate on the experience. Often, this method was successful in drawing out participants' own views and values, which emerged while carefully disentangling the challenges they had faced. Future research may combine blinded topics or questions with some questions that participants reflect on prior to the interview so that participants feel less pressured by the time constraints.

Another limitation from the methods applied during this study is the development of the interview guide and use of topics from the literature review. The topics covered in this study, namely HIV/AIDS, women's enrolment in research and the role of Islamic scholars, were pre-determined. It is pertinent to consider whether the inclusion of these topics influenced the responses of participants and subsequent analysis, or whether these are real issues for researchers in these contexts. During my interviews, I carefully began the discussion with open questions and probed based on the responses of participants. There were a range of other issues that emerged from the interviews. However, the four cross-cutting themes were chosen because they emerged as being important from the literature review and analysis of the earlier interviews, and they were areas appropriate for considering whether and how Islam influences biomedical research ethics. These themes also helped to relate the data and discussion from this research to broader bioethical discussions around universal versus relative ethical principles and moral particularism (see Chapters 1 and 7).

Given such limitations, the conclusions drawn about the case study sites, Malaysia and Iran, may not be generalised to other countries. Despite such limitations, it is hoped that the methods and findings within this research will be a starting point for future research in a nascent area of study.

Conclusions

In summary, this chapter details the rationale for the empirical study; the theoretical and practical foundations of the chosen research design; the methods employed during the various stages of the study, including study site selection, recruitment, data collection and analysis and the advantages and disadvantages of each of these. This chapter also outlines some of the ethical concerns that arose during my fieldwork, and how these were prepared for and/or addressed. It also presents an account of how I reflected on my role as a researcher to ensure reflexivity and objectivity. It accounts for my pre-existing values and experiences and how they may have impacted the data collection and analysis. The chapter also summarizes the process of data analysis, including an ethical analysis of respondents' views as well as the process of developing the four key themes around which the data chapters are arranged. Finally the chapter provides a detailed account of the limitations of this study in the hope that future researchers can develop strategies to overcome these and/or employ alternative methods.

Bibliography

Ansari, A. (2014). *Iran: A very short introduction*. Oxford: Oxford University Press.
Axworthy, M. (2010). *A history of Iran: Empire of the mind*. London: Basic Books.
Beauchamp, T. L. & Childress, J. F. (2001). *Principles of biomedical ethics*. New York: Oxford University Press.
Bourdieu, P. (2004). *Science of science and reflexivity*. Cambridge, UK: Polity.
Chenail, R. J. (1995). Presenting qualitative data. *The Qualitative Report*, 2(3), 1–9.
Crowe, S., Cresswell, K., Robertson, A., Huby, G., Avery, A. & Sheikh, A. (2011). The case study approach. *BMC Med Res Methodol*, 11, 100. doi:10.1186/1471-2288-11-100.

Delvoie, L. A. & Ansari, A. M. (2001). Iran, Islam, and democracy: The politics of managing change. *International Journal*, 56(4), 699. doi:10.2307/40203613.

Denscombe, M. (2014). *The good research guide: For small-scale social research projects.* Maidenhead, UK: McGraw-Hill Education.

Drabble, J. H. & Booth, A. (2000). *An economic history of Malaysia, c.1800–1990: The transition to modern economic growth.* Basingstoke, UK: Palgrave Macmillan.

El-Menouar, Y. & Stiftung, B. (2014). The five dimensions of Muslim religiosity: Results of an empirical study. *Methods, data, analyses*, 8(1), 53–78.

Emanuel, E. J., Wendler, D. & Grady, C. (2000). What makes clinical research ethical?. *JAMA*, 283(20), 2701–2711.

Entessar, N. (1988). Criminal law and the legal system in revolutionary Iran. *BC Third World LJ*, 8, 91.

Gale, N. K., Heath, G., Cameron, E., Rashid, S. & Redwood, S. (2013). Using the framework method for the analysis of qualitative data in multi-disciplinary health research. *BMC Medical Research Methodology*, 13(1), 117. doi:10.1186/1471-2288-13-117.

Garrafa, V., Solbakk, J. H., Vidal, S. & Lorenzo, C. (2010). Between the needy and the greedy: The quest for a just and fair ethics of clinical research. *Journal of Medical Ethics*, 36(8), 500–504. doi:10.1136/jme.2009.032656.

Gheissair, A., Nasr, V. & Nasr, S. V. R. (2009). *Democracy in Iran: History and the quest for liberty.* New York: Oxford University Press.

Glickman, S. W., McHutchison, J. G., Peterson, E. D., Cairns, C. B., Harrington, R. A., Califf, R. M. & Schulman, K. A. (2009). Ethical and scientific implications of the globalization of clinical research. *New England Journal of Medicine*, 360(8), 816–823. doi:10.1056/nejmsb0803929.

Green, J., Thorogood, N. & Green, G. (2013). *Qualitative methods for health research (Introducing qualitative methods series)* (2nd ed.). Los Angeles, CA: SAGE Publications.

Gross, A. & Hirose, M. (2007). Conducting clinical trials in Asia. http://www.pacific bridgemedical.com/publications/asia/2007_conducting_clinical_trials (Last accessed 20 August 2016).

Guest, G., Bunce, A. & Johnson, L. (2006). How many interviews are enough? An experiment with data saturation and variability. *Field methods*, 18(1), 59–82.

Hobbs, D. & Wright, R. (Eds.). (2006). *The SAGE handbook of fieldwork.* London: SAGE.

Hock, S. S. (2007). *The population of Malaysia.* Singapore: Institute of Southeast Asian Studies.

Hodgson, M. G. S. (1977a). *The venture of Islam: Conscience and history in a world civilization. Volume 1: The classical age of Islam.* Chicago, IL: University of Chicago Press.

Hodgson, M. G. S. (1977b). *The venture of Islam: Conscience and history in a world civilization. Volume 2: The expansion of Islam in the middle periods* (2nd ed.). Chicago, IL: University of Chicago Press.

Hooker, V. M. & Osborne, M. E. (2003). *A short history of Malaysia: Linking east and west.* Crows Nest, Australia: Allen & Unwin.

Huber, S. & Huber, O. W. (2012). The centrality of religiosity scale (CRS). *Religions*, 3(4), 710–724. doi:10.3390/rel3030710.

Imam, S. S., Nurullah, A. S., Makol-Abdul, P. R., Rahman, S. A. & Noon, H. M. (2009). Spiritual and psychological health of Malaysian youths. In R. L. Piedmont & A. Village (Eds.) *Research in the social scientific study of religion*, 20 (pp. 85–102). Leiden, The Netherlands: Brill.

Kamali, M. H. (1997). Islamic law in Malaysia: Issues and developments. *Yearbook of Islamic and Middle Eastern Law Online*, 4(1), 153–179.

Korieth, K. & Anderson, A. (2013). New growth and decline in Asia clinical trials. *The Center Watch Monthly*, 20, 1–6.

Larijani, B. & Zahedi, F. (2008). Contemporary medical ethics: an overview from Iran. *Developing World Bioethics*, 8(3), 192–196.

Larijani, B.Zahedi, F. & Malek-Afzali, H. (2005). Medical ethics in the Islamic Republic of Iran. *East Mediterr Health J*, 11(5–6), 1061–1072.

Larijani, B., Zahedi, F., Nouri, M., Bagheri, A., Heshmat, R., Motevaseli, E. & Malekafzali, H. (2006). Ethics committees and externally-sponsored research in Iran. *Journal of Medical Ethics and History of Medicine*, (Suppl. 1), 1–6.

Mir-Hosseini, Z. (2010). Sharia and national law in Iran. In J. M. Otto (Ed.). *Sharia incorporated: A comparative overview of the legal systems of twelve Muslim countries in past and present* (pp. 319–372). Leiden, The Netherlands: Leiden University Press.

Padela, A. I. (2013a). Islamic bioethics: Between sacred law, lived experiences, and state authority. *Theoretical Medicine and Bioethics*, 34(2), 65–80. doi:10.1007/s11017-013-9249-1.

Pope, C., Ziebland, S. & Mays, N. (2000). Analysing qualitative data. *Bmj*, 320(7227), 114–116.

Ritchie, J. & Lewis, J. (Eds.). (2003). *Qualitative research practice: A guide for social science students and researchers*. London: SAGE Publications.

Sachedina, A. (2009). *Islamic biomedical ethics: Principles and application*. New York: Oxford University Press.

Sandelowski, M. (1994). Focus on qualitative methods: The use of quotes in qualitative research. *Research in nursing & health*, 17(6), 479–482.

Sandelowski, M. (1998). Writing a good read: Strategies for re-presenting qualitative data. *Research in Nursing & Health*, 21(4), 375–382.

Setia, A. (2007). Three meanings of Islamic science: Toward operationalizing Islamization of science. *Islam and Science*, 5(1), 23–52.

Shuaib, F. S. (2012). The Islamic legal system in Malaysia, *Pac. Rim L. & Pol'y J.*, 21, 85.

Silverman, D. (2013). *Doing qualitative research: A practical handbook* (4th ed.). Thousand Oaks, CA: SAGE Publications.

Smith, J., Bekker, H. & Cheater, F. (2011). Theoretical versus pragmatic design in qualitative research. *Nurse Researcher*, 18(2), 39–51. doi:10.7748/nr2011.01.18.2.39.c8283.

Stake, R. (2000). Case studies. In N. Denzin & Y. Lincoln (Eds.). *Handbook of qualitative research* (2nd ed.) (pp. 435–454). Thousand Oaks, CA: SAGE.

Tan, A. K. G., Dunn, R. A., Samad, M. I. A. & Feisul, M. I. (2010). Sociodemographic and health-lifestyle determinants of obesity risks in Malaysia. *Asia-Pacific Journal of Public Health*, 23(2), 192–202. doi:10.1177/1010539509359535.

Tremayne, S. (2009). Law, ethics and donor technologies in Shia Iran. In D. Birenbaum-Carmeli & M. C. Inhorn (Eds.). *Assisting reproduction, testing genes: Global encounters with the new Biotechnologies* (pp. 144–163). Oxford: Berghahn Books.

Winter, T. (Ed.). (2008). *The Cambridge companion to classical Islamic theology (Cambridge companions to religion)* (3rd ed.). Cambridge: Cambridge University Press.

Yusuf, A. (2014). Ethical issues in research ethics governance and their application to the Malaysian context. DPhil thesis. University of Oxford.

Zahedi, F. & Larijani, B. (2008). National bioethical legislation and guidelines for biomedical research in the Islamic Republic of Iran. *Bulletin of the World Health Organization*, 86(8), 630–634.

Zali, M. R., Shahraz, S. & Borzabadi, S. (2002). Bioethics in Iran: Legislation as the main problem. *Arch Iranian Med* 5(3), 136–140.

Appendix

Draft interview guide for semi-structured, in-depth interviews with scholars, guideline developers, REC members, principle investigators and fieldworkers

Part A: Introduction and a brief description of what the research is about

a. What is your experience of clinical research?

    i   To begin with, could you please tell me a little about yourself, how you got into this role and what you do?

b. What kinds of difficult decisions do you face in your work?

    i   What kinds of difficult questions do you face in your work?
    ii To what extent do you think these are ethical/moral questions?
    iii I am interested in ethics and ethical problems, but this isn't a term everyone uses.

c. What resources do you have/use to navigate through such questions? Are there guidelines/laws?

Part B: Islam as personal faith

d. Does your faith (or the faith of others) influence what you consider to be an ethical/moral problem?

    i   What role does your or your participants' faith play in your work?
    ii I am interested in the role of faith and research; so I want to know from you, how does faith feature in your work – your faith and/or the faith of others?
    iii From what you have described, does your faith influence why you consider these problems as moral/ethical problems? Why? Why not?

e. Do you think faith is important in defining what an ethical/problem is, in the context of research?

    i   Do you think it is important to consider Islamic values or the Muslim context when thinking about clinical research? What problems may arise when these are moral/ethical questions?

ii   Some people have told me that Islam is important in their private lives, but when they are at work their decisions are governed by professional codes of ethics and laws. What do you think about this?

f. Is it necessary to consider faith when ensuring that research is conducted ethically? Why? Why not?

i   Is faith a consideration when determining what is ethically acceptable research where you work? Why? Why not? Do you agree with this? Why? Why not?

ii   If faith is a necessary consideration, then what do you think are the challenges and priorities for the future in ensuring that research is conducted ethically within a Muslim community like yours, whilst also ensuring respect for religious plurality and freedoms?

Part C: Institutional aspects of Islam and their authority

g. What role, if any, does Islam play in the national law and national prioritisation for health and health research?

i   Is this role of Islam through a national council, laws, or consultation?

ii   Why is it considered important/relevant for your context?"

h. What do you understand by the term "Islamic ethics"?

i   What are the sources, principles and implications for research?

ii   What do you think the Islamic view is on clinical research?

i. Does Islam's institutional aspects impact research priorities, research guideline production and research conduct? If so, how? If not, why not?

i   Is there religious representation within the ethics committee? If so, why? Why not?

ii   Have you had to consult a *fatwah* council/religious authority within an ethics committee/the conduct of research?

iii   Is the choice of research topics determined by a scholarly or textual analysis? If so, how? If not, why not?"

iv   Are ethical principles influenced by an Islamic framework?

v   Should researchers and fieldworkers implement Islamic teaching in their work?

vi   Why, in your opinion, has there been such a focus on topics within the Islamic ethical discourse and very little focus on the conduct of research trials?

j. Have you noticed changes in how Islam influences health research and ethics over the course of your career?

k. How is the role of Islam changing in the area of emerging technologies? How do you envision its role in the future?

l. **In your opinion, what is the role of Islam in bioethics/research ethics?**

   i   How much is it for maintaining culture?
   ii A religious necessity?
   iii Or, a distinct means of practical deliberation?

Part D: Global health, bioethics and Muslim contexts

m. **What do you understand by the term "secular ethics"? What are your views about secular ethical principles, and how do they impact biomedical research?**

   i   For example, do you share the values set out in Beauchamp and Childress's work as well as guidelines, such as Helsinki and CIOMS? Do you think you "should" share them?
   ii Many of the challenges/questions people mention to me are more general ethical considerations, rather than issues that are rooted in faith, e.g., benefits and harms. Does this mean that faith only influences very specific ethical issues, e.g., ones to do with culture (women's consent) or religious practice (fasting, m-f relations)? What do you understand by the term *benefit and harm*? And does faith influence the understanding of such "universal" ethical principles? If so, how?
   iii What is your understanding of autonomy and confidentiality – do you consider such values as universally shared? What about views on public over private interests in Muslim contexts? Is this relevant in your work?

n. **When there is an international collaboration, how does the collaboration impact on what is defined as an ethical problem, and how are such problems addressed?**

   i   Does faith need to be considered in such collaborations? If so, why and to what extent? Does this consideration take place? Why? Why not?

Part E: Case studies of particular issues in research ethics

o. **In the literature and during my discussion with others, it has been mentioned that there are certain types of research that cannot be done in Muslim contexts, e.g., looking at the efficacy of HIV prevention programmes using contraception, as this promotes promiscuity in the society. Have you ever come across this or other such issues, and could you tell me more about these?**

   i   What is the underlying cause of such concerns? Is it religious? If so, what are the sources/explanations? Or, is it culture? If so, why is such an issue culturally important/sensitive?

p. **What are your views on:**

   i   Female consent – Some people suggest that Muslim women should be co-consented with their husbands, especially if that is what the woman/

community expects. What do you think about this? Why? (REF paper from Malaysia)

ii Consent of pregnant woman – Some authors have suggested that a husband's consent is necessary when enrolling a pregnant woman into a study. What do you think about this? Why? (REF IOMS, paper from Malaysia, country guidelines, e.g., Saudi, Qatar)

iii Sharing of genetic material and benefits – Some people say that the benefits and samples from genetic studies should not be shared with other countries that have different value systems. How does collaborative work happen here, and what do you think about the sharing of genetic material with other countries?

iv Use of impure ingredients in trial interventions, e.g., vaccines – Is this a problem? If so, why? Why not?

v Gender relations, e.g., male/female research and participants – Is this a problem? If so, why? Why not?

vi Storage of blood, genetic data and tissue – Is this a problem? If so, why? Why not?

vii How does faith and/or culture influence your views on i-vi above. Can faith and culture be considered distinct regarding such issues? Why? Why not?

q. Does the "Muslim majority" context make a difference?

i When people train in regions/countries where, as a Muslim, they are a minority, is there a difference in the way they approach the question of how being Muslim or Islam influences their decision making?

ii When they are a minority, do they have to feel more strongly about certain issues to preserve their notion of what is (Islamically) right because there is no institutional support for it?

Other details about the interviewing process and criteria are available from the author on request.

Bibliography

Abou Bakr, O. (2015). The interpretative legacy of Qiwamah as an exegetical construct. In Z. Mir-Hosseini, M. Al-Sharmani & J. Rumminger (Eds.). *Men in charge?: Rethinking authority in Muslim legal tradition* (pp. 44–62). London: Oneworld Publications.

Adamson, P. (2015). *Philosophy in the Islamic world: A very short introduction*. Oxford: Oxford University Press.

Afifi, R. Y. (2007). Biomedical research ethics: An Islamic view. Part II. *International Journal of Surgery*, 5(6), 381–383.

Aghajanian, A. & Merhyar, A. H. (1999). Fertility, contraceptive use and family planning program activity in the Islamic Republic of Iran. *International Family Planning Perspectives*, 25(2), 98–102.

Ahmed, A. & Suleman, M. (2018). Islamic perspectives on the genome and the human person: Why the soul matters. In M. Ghaly (Ed.). *Islamic ethics and the genome question* (pp. 139–168). Brill.

Aksoy, S. & Elmali, A. (2002). Core concepts of the Four Principles of Bioethics as found in Islamic tradition. *Med. & L.*, 21, 211.

Aksoy, S. & Tenik, A. (2002). The "four principles of bioethics" as found in 13th century Muslim scholar Mawlana's teachings. *BMC Medical Ethics*, 3(1). doi:10.1186/1472-6939-3-4.

Alahmad, G., Al-Jumah, M. & Dierickx, K. (2012). Review of national research ethics regulations and guidelines in middle eastern Arab countries. *BMC Medical Ethics*, 13(1). doi:10.1186/1472-6939-13-34.

Al-Bar, M. A. & Chamsi-Pasha, H. (2015). *Contemporary bioethics: Islamic perspective*. New York: Springer.

Al-Hibri, A. Y. (1997). Islam, law and custom: Redefining Muslim women's rights. *American University Journal of International Law and Policy*, 12(1), 1. http://scholarship.richmond.edu/cgi/viewcontent.cgi?article=1157&context=law-faculty-publications (Last accessed 19 August 2016).

Al-Jumah, M., Abolfotouh, M. A., Alabdulkareem, I. B., Balkhy, H. H., Al-Jeraisy, M. I., Al-Swaid, A. F. & Al-Knawy, B. (2011). Public attitude towards biomedical research at outpatient clinics of King Abdulaziz medical city, Riyadh, Saudi Arabia. *Eastern Mediterranean Health Journal*, 17(6), 536.

Annas, G. J. & Grodin, M. A. (2008). The Nuremberg Code. In E. J. Emanuel, C. C. Grady, R. A. Crouch, R. K. Lie, F. G. Miller & D. D. Wendler (Eds.). *The Oxford textbook of clinical research ethics* (pp. 136–140). New York: Oxford University Press.

Ansari, A. (2014). *Iran: A very short introduction*. Oxford: Oxford University Press.

Arksey, H. & O'Malley, L. (2005). Scoping studies: Towards a methodological framework. *International Journal of Social Research Methodology*, 8(1), 19–32.

Atighetchi, D. (2007). *Islamic bioethics: Problems and perspectives.* Dordrecht, The Netherlands: Springer.

Axworthy, M. (2010). *A history of Iran: Empire of the mind.* London: Basic Books.

Bagheri, A. (2014). Priority setting in Islamic bioethics: Top 10 bioethical challenges in Islamic countries. *Asian Bioethics Review*, 6(4), 391–401. doi:10.1353/asb.2014.0031.

Banu az-Zubair, M. K. (2007). Who is a parent? Parenthood in Islamic ethics. *Journal of Medical Ethics*, 33(10), 605–609. doi:10.1136/jme.2005.015396.

Barmania, S. & Aljunid, S. M. (2016). Navigating HIV prevention policy and Islam in Malaysia: Contention, compatibility or reconciliation? Findings from in-depth interviews among key stakeholders. *BMC Public Health*, 16(1), 524.

Berlinguer, G. (2004). Bioethics, health and inequality. *The Lancet*, 364(9439), 1086–1091. doi:10.1016/s0140-6736(04)17066-9.

Beauchamp, T. L. & Childress, J. F. (2001). *Principles of biomedical ethics.* New York: Oxford University Press.

Bhutta, Z. A. (2002). Ethics in international health research: A perspective from the developing world. *Bulletin of the World Health Organization*, 80(2), 114–120.

Blum, L. A. (1994). *Moral perception and particularity.* Cambridge: Cambridge University Press.

Bourdieu, P. (2004). *Science of science and reflexivity.* Cambridge: Polity.

Bracanovic, T. (2010). Respect for cultural diversity in bioethics. Empirical, conceptual and normative constraints. *Medicine, Health Care and Philosophy*, 14(3), 229–236. doi:10.1007/s11019-010-9299-3.

Brockopp, J. E. & Eich, T. (2008). *Muslim medical ethics: From theory to practice.* University of South Carolina Press.

Brody, H. & Macdonald, A. (2013). Religion and bioethics: Toward an expanded understanding. *Theoretical Medicine and Bioethics*, 34(2), 133–145. doi:10.1007/s11017-013-9244-6.

Caballero, B. (2002). Ethical issues for collaborative research in developing countries. *The American Journal of Clinical Nutrition*, 76(4), 717–720.

Carter, B. J. (2010). Removing the offending member: Iran and the sex-change or die option as the alternative to the death sentencing of homosexuals. *J. Gender Race & Just.*, 14, 797–832.

Chattopadhyay, S. & De Vries, R. (2012). Respect for cultural diversity in bioethics is an ethical imperative. *Medicine, Health Care and Philosophy*, 16(4), 639–645. doi:10.1007/s11019-012-9433-5.

Chenail, R. J. (1995). Presenting qualitative data. *The Qualitative Report*, 2(3), 1–9.

Childress, J. F. (2009). Forward. In A. Sachedina (Ed.). *Islamic biomedical ethics: Principles and application* (p. viii). New York: Oxford University Press.

CIOMS. (2002). International ethical guidelines for biomedical research involving human subjects. www.fhi360.org/training/fr/retc/pdf_files/cioms.pdf (Last accessed 15 January 2020).

Clausen, C. (1996). Welcome to post-culturalism. *The American Scholar*, 65(3), 379–388.

Colquhoun, H. L., Levac, D., O'Brien, K. K., Straus, S., Tricco, A. C., Perrier, L., Kastner, M. & Moher, D. (2014). Scoping reviews: Time for clarity in definition, methods, and reporting. *Journal of clinical epidemiology*, 67(12), 1291–1294.

Curran, W. J. (1973). The Tuskegee syphilis study. *New England Journal of Medicine*, 289 (14), 730–731. doi:10.1056/nejm197310042891406.

Crowe, S., Cresswell, K., Robertson, A., Huby, G., Avery, A. & Sheikh, A. (2011). The case study approach. *BMC Med Res Methodol*, 11, 100. doi:10.1186/1471-2288-11-100.

Dancy, J. (2004). *Ethics without principles*. Oxford: Oxford University Press on Demand.

Darley, J. M. & Latane, B. (1968). Bystander intervention in emergencies: Diffusion of responsibility. *J Pers Soc Psychol*, 8(4), 377–383.

Dawson, C. (2013). *Religion and culture*. Washington, DC: CUA Press.

Delvoie, L. A. & Ansari, A. M. (2001). Iran, Islam and democracy: The politics of managing change. *International Journal*, 56(4), 699. doi:10.2307/40203613.

Denscombe, M. (2014). *The good research guide: For small-scale social research projects*. Maidenhead, UK: McGraw-Hill Education.

Drabble, J. H. & Booth, A. (2000). *An economic history of Malaysia, c.1800–1990: The transition to modern economic growth*. Basingstoke, UK: Palgrave Macmillan.

Duffy, M. F. (1988). The challenge to the Christian community. *Religious Education*, 83 (2), 190–199.

Dunn, M., Sheehan, M., Hope, T. & Parker, M. (2012). Toward methodological innovation in empirical ethics research. *Cambridge Quarterly of Healthcare Ethics*, 21(04), 466–480.

Durante, C. (2008). Bioethics in a pluralistic society: Bioethical methodology in lieu of moral diversity. *Medicine, Health Care and Philosophy*, 12(1), 35–47. doi:10.1007/s11019-008-9148-9.

El Fadl, K. A. (2014). *Speaking in God's name: Islamic law, authority and women*. Oxford: Oneworld Publications.

El-Hazmi, M. A. (2003). Ethics of genetic counseling. Basic concepts and relevance to Islamic communities. *Annals of Saudi medicine*, 24(2), 84–92.

Ellsberg, M., Heise, L., Pena, R., Agurto, S. & Winkvist, A. (2001). Researching domestic violence against women: Methodological and ethical considerations. *Stud Fam Plann*, 32(1), 1–16.

El-Menouar, Y. & Stiftung, B. (2014). The five dimensions of Muslim religiosity: Results of an empirical study. *Methods, data, analyses*, 8(1), 53–78.

Emanuel, E. J., Grady, C. C., Crouch, R. A., Lie, R. K., Miller, F. G. & Wendler, D. D. (Eds.). (2008). *The Oxford textbook of clinical research ethics*. Oxford: Oxford University Press.

Emanuel, E. J., Wendler, D. & Grady, C. (2000). What makes clinical research ethical?. *JAMA*, 283(20), 2701–2711.

Emanuel, E. J., Wendler, D., Killen, J. & Grady, C. (2004). What makes clinical research in developing countries ethical? The benchmarks of ethical research. *The Journal of Infectious Diseases*, 189(5), 930–937. doi:10.1086/381709.

Engelhardt, H. T. (1996). *The foundations of bioethics*. Oxford: Oxford University Press.

Engelhardt, H. T. (2000). *The foundations of Christian bioethics*. Lisse, The Netherlands: Swets & Zeitlinger.

Entessar, N. (1988). Criminal law and the legal system in revolutionary Iran. *BC Third World LJ*, 8, 91.

Fadel, H. E. (2010). Ethics of clinical research: An Islamic perspective. *Journal of the Islamic Medical Association of North America*, 42(2).

Fakhry, M. (1991). *Ethical theories in Islam*, (8). Leiden, The Netherlands: Brill.

Fakhry, M. (2009). *Islamic philosophy: A beginner's guide*. London: Oneworld Publications.

Farrell, M. (2003). Condoms and AIDS Prevention: A comparison of three faith-based organizations in Uganda. *AIDS and Anthropology Bulletin*, 15(3).

FIMA. (2015). About FIMA. http://fimaweb.net/cms/index.php/about. (Last accessed 22 August 2016).

FIMA Admin. (2015). FIMA declaration on global efforts to combat the HIV/AIDS pandemic. https://fimaweb.net/fima-declaration-on-global-efforts-to-combat-the-hiv-aids-pandemic (Last accessed 22 August 2016).

Forsythe, S., Rau, B., Alrutz, N., Gold, E., Hayman, J. & Lux, L. (1996). *AIDS in Kenya: Socioeconomic impact and policy implications.* www.popline.org/node/301833 (Last accessed 7 May 2017).

Freedman, B. (1987). Scientific value and validity as ethical requirements for research: A proposed Explication. *IRB: Ethics and Human Research,* 9(6), 7. doi:10.2307/3563623.

Frieden, T. R. & Collins, F. S. (2010). Intentional infection of vulnerable populations in 1946–48. *JAMA,* 304(18). doi:10.1001/jama.2010.1554.

Gale, N. K., Heath, G., Cameron, E., Rashid, S. & Redwood, S. (2013). Using the framework method for the analysis of qualitative data in multi-disciplinary health research. *BMC Medical Research Methodology,* 13(1), 117. doi:10.1186/1471-2288-13-117.

Garcia-Moreno, C., Jansen, H. A., Ellsberg, M., Heise, L. & Watts, C. H. (2006). Prevalence of intimate partner violence: Findings from the WHO multi-country study on women's health and domestic violence. *The Lancet,* 368(9543), 1260–1269.

Garrafa, V., Solbakk, J. H., Vidal, S. & Lorenzo, C. (2010). Between the needy and the greedy: The quest for a just and fair ethics of clinical research. *Journal of Medical Ethics,* 36(8), 500–504. doi:10.1136/jme.2009.032656.

Garrard, E. & Wilkinson, S. (2005). Mind the gap: The use of empirical evidence in bioethics. In M. Häyry, T. Takala & P. Herissone-Kelly (Eds.). *Bioethics and social reality* (pp. 77–92). Amsterdam, The Netherlands: Rodopi.

Gatrad, A. R. & Sheikh, A. (2001). Medical ethics and Islam: Principles and practice. *Archives of Disease in Childhood,* 84(1), 72–75.

Ghaly, M. (2012). The beginning of human life: Islamic bioethical perspectives. *Zygon®,* 47(1), 175–213.

Ghaly, M. (2013a). Collective religio-scientific discussions on Islam and HIV/AIDS: I. Biomedical scientists. *Zygon®,* 48(3), 671–708.

Ghaly, M. (2013b). Islamic bioethics in the twenty-first century. *Zygon®,* 48(3), 592–599.

Ghaly, M. (2015). Biomedical scientists as co-muftis: Their contribution to contemporary Islamic bioethics. *Die Welt des Islams,* 55(3–4), 286–311.

Gheissair, A., Nasr, V. & Nasr, S. V. R. (2009). *Democracy in Iran: History and the quest for liberty.* New York: Oxford University Press.

Glickman, S. W., McHutchison, J. G., Peterson, E. D., Cairns, C. B., Harrington, R. A., Califf, R. M. & Schulman, K. A. (2009). Ethical and scientific implications of the globalization of clinical research. *New England Journal of Medicine,* 360(8), 816–823. doi:10.1056/nejmsb0803929.

Global Forum for Health Research (2004). *The 10/90 report on health research, 2003–2004.* Switzerland: Global Forum for Health Research.

Green, J., Thorogood, N. & Green, G. (2013). *Qualitative methods for health research (Introducing qualitative methods series)* (2nd ed.). Los Angeles, CA: SAGE Publications.

Gross, A. & Hirose, M. (2007). Conducting clinical trials in Asia. www.pacificbridgemedical.com/publications/asia/2007_conducting_clinical_trials (Last accessed 20 August 2016).

Guest, G., Bunce, A. & Johnson, L. (2006). How many interviews are enough? An experiment with data saturation and variability. *Field methods,* 18(1), 59–82.

Hallaq, W. B. (2009). *Shar⬚'a: Theory, practice, transformations*. Cambridge: Cambridge University Press.

Hamdy, S. (2012). *Our bodies belong to God: Organ transplants, Islam, and the struggle for human dignity in Egypt*. University of California Press.

Hasnain, M. (2005). Cultural approach to HIV/AIDS harm reduction in Muslim countries. *Harm Reduction Journal*, 2(1), 1.

Hobbs, D. & Wright, R. (Eds.). (2006). *The SAGE handbook of fieldwork*. London: SAGE.

Hock, S. S. (2007). *The population of Malaysia*. Singapore: Institute of Southeast Asian Studies.

Hodgson, M. G. S. (1977a). *The venture of Islam: Conscience and history in a world civilization. Volume 1: The classical age of Islam*. Chicago, IL: University of Chicago Press.

Hodgson, M. G. S. (1977b). *The venture of Islam: Conscience and history in a world civilization. Volume 2: The expansion of Islam in the middle periods* (2nd ed.). Chicago, IL: University of Chicago Press.

Hooker, V. M. & Osborne, M. E. (2003). *A short history of Malaysia: Linking east and west*. Crows Nest, Australia: Allen & Unwin.

Hourani, G. F. (2007). *Reason and tradition in Islamic ethics*. Cambridge University Press.

HRH The Prince of Wales. (2007). Foreword. In A. Sheikh & A. R. Gatrad (Eds.). *Caring for Muslim patients*. New York: Radcliffe Publishing.

Huber, S. & Huber, O. W. (2012). The centrality of religiosity scale (CRS). *Religions*, 3 (4), 710–724. doi:10.3390/rel3030710.

Ibn Majah. Book 31, Hadith 3436. *Sunan Ibn Majah*. http://sunnah.com/ibnmajah/31 (Retrieved 23 August 2016).

Ilkilic, I. (2002). Bioethical conflicts between Muslim patients and German physicians and the principles of biomedical ethics. *Med. & L.*, 21(2), 243–256.

Ilsselmuiden, C. B., Kass, N. E., Sewankambo, K. N. & Lavery, J. V. (2010). Evolving values in ethics and global health research. *Global Public Health*, 5(2), 154–163. doi:10.1080/17441690903436599.

Imam, S. S., Nurullah, A. S., Makol-Abdul, P. R., Rahman, S. A. & Noon, H. M. (2009). Spiritual and psychological health of Malaysian youths. In R. L. Piedmont and A. Village (Eds.). *Research in the social scientific study of religion*, 20 (pp. 85–102). Leiden, The Netherlands: Brill.

Inhorn, M. C. (2008). Conclusion. In J. E. Brockopp & T. Eich (Eds.). *Muslim medical ethics: From theory to practice* (pp. 252–256). Columbia, SC: University of South Carolina Press.

Inhorn, M. C. (2012). *Local babies, global science: Gender, religion, and in vitro fertilization in Egypt*. New York: Routledge.

Inhorn, M. C. & Serour, G. I. (2011). Islam, medicine, and Arab-Muslim refugee health in America after 9/11. *The Lancet*, 378(9794), 935–943. doi:10.1016/s0140-6736(11) 61041-6.

IOMS (Islamic Organization for Medical Sciences). (2004). International Conference on "Islamic Code of Medical Ethics". http://islamset.net/ioms/code2004/index.html (Last accessed 15 January 2020).

IOMS (Islamic Organization for Medical Sciences). (2005). International ethical guidelines for biomedical research involving human subjects "an Islamic perspective". In A. R. El-Gendy & A. R. A. Al-Awadi (Eds.). *The international Islamic code for medical and health ethics* (Vol. 2, 121–276). Kuwait: Islamic Organization for Medical Sciences.

Ives, J. & Dunn, M. (2010). Who's arguing?: A call for reflexivity in bioethics. *Bioethics*, 24 (5), 256–265.

Ives, J., Dunn, M. & Cribb, A. (Eds.). (2016). *Empirical bioethics: Theoretical and practical perspectives* (Vol. 37). Cambridge: Cambridge University Press.

Jonsen, A. R. (1998). *The birth of bioethics*. Oxford: Oxford University Press.

Kagimu, M., Marum, E., Wabwire-Mangen, F., Nakyanjo, N., Walakira, Y. & Hogle, J. (1998). Evaluation of the effectiveness of AIDS health education intervention in the Muslim community in Uganda. *AIDS Education and Prevention*, 10(3), 215–228.

Kamali, M. H. (1997). Islamic law in Malaysia: Issues and developments. *Yearbook of Islamic and Middle Eastern Law Online*, 4(1), 153–179.

Kamali, M. H. (2008). *Maqasid Al-Shariah made simple*. London: IIIT.

Kamarulzaman, A. & Saifuddeen, S. M. (2010). Islam and harm reduction. *International Journal of Drug Policy*, 21(2), 115–118.

Kaur, S. (2011). *The adequacy of the ethics review process in Malaysia: Protection of the interests of mentally incapacitated adults who enrol in clinical trials*. Doctor of Philosophy thesis. University College London. http://discovery.ucl.ac.uk/1324539/1/1324539.pdf (Last accessed 4 January 2015).

Kazim, F. (2007). Critical analysis of the Pakistan Medical Dental Council code and bioethical issues. Master's Thesis in Applied Ethics. Linköpings Universitet, Sweden. Centre for Applied Ethics. www.diva-portal.org/smash/get/diva2:23919/FULLTEXT01.pdf (Last accessed 29 April 2016).

Kennedy, D. (2007). Gays should be hanged, says Iranian minister. *The Times*. www.timesonline.co.uk/tol/news/world/middle-east/article2859606.ece (Last accessed 22 August 2016).

Kerasidou, A. & Parker, M. (2014). Does science need bioethicists? Ethics and science collaboration in biomedical research. *Research Ethics*, 10(4), 214–226. doi:10.1177/1747016114554252.

Kermani, F. (2010). How to run clinical trials in the Middle East. *SCRIP*(February), 1–8.

Keyserlingk, E. W. (1993). Ethics codes and guidelines for health care and research: Can respect for autonomy be a multi-cultural principle. In J. R. Coombs & E. Winkler (Eds.). *Applied ethics: A reader* (pp. 319–415). Oxford: Blackwell Publishers.

Kingori, P. (2013). Experiencing everyday ethics in context: Frontline data collectors perspectives and practices of bioethics. *Social Science & Medicine*, 98, 361–370. doi:10.1016/j.socscimed.2013.10.013.

Kleinman, A. (1999). Moral experience and ethical reflection: Can ethnography reconcile them? A quandary for "the new bioethics". *Daedalus*, 128(4), 69–97.

Kon, A. A. (2009). The role of empirical research in bioethics. *The American Journal of Bioethics*, 9(6–7),59–65. doi:10.1080/15265160902874320.

Korieth, K. & Anderson, A. (2013). New growth and decline in Asia clinical trials. *The Center Watch Monthly*, 20, 1–6.

Kyriakides-Yeldham, A. (2005). Islamic medical ethics and the straight path of God. *Islam and Christian–Muslim Relations*, 16(3), 213–225.

Lagarde, E., Pison, G. & Enel, C. (1998). Risk behaviours and AIDS knowledge in a rural community of Senegal: Relationship with sources of AIDS information. *International Journal of Epidemiology*, 27(5), 890–896.

Lairumbi, G. M., Parker, M., Fitzpatrick, R. & English, M. C. (2011). Stakeholders understanding of the concept of benefit sharing in health research in Kenya: A qualitative study. *BMC Medical Ethics*, 12(1). doi:10.1186/1472-6939-12-20.

Larijani, B. & Zahedi, F. (2007). Biotechnology, bioethics and national ethical guidelines in biomedical research in Iran. *Asian Biotechnology and Development Review*, 9(3), 43–56.

Larijani, B. & Zahedi, F. (2008). Contemporary medical ethics: An overview from Iran. *Developing World Bioethics*, 8(3), 192–196.

Larijani, B., Zahedi, F. & Malek-Afzali, H. (2005). Medical ethics in the Islamic Republic of Iran. *East Mediterr Health J*, 11(5–6), 1061–1072.

Larijani, B., Zahedi, F., Nouri, M., Bagheri, A., Heshmat, R., Motevaseli, E. & Malekafzali, H. (2006). Ethics committees and externally-sponsored research in Iran. *Journal of Medical Ethics and History of Medicine*, (Suppl. 1), 1–6.

Leget, C., Borry, P. & De Vries, R. (2009). "Nobody Tosses a Dwarf!" The relation between the empirical and the normative reexamined. *Bioethics*, 23(4), 226–235.

Lin, V. (1997). Resource review. Investing in health research and development: Report of the ad hoc committee on health research relating to future intervention options. World Health Organization, Geneva, 1996. *Health Promotion International*, 12(4), 331–332. doi:10.1093/heapro/12.4.331.

Lings, M. (2012). *Muhammad: His life based on the earliest sources*. Cambridge: Islamic Texts Society.

Lurie, P. & Wolfe, S. M. (1997). Unethical trials of interventions to reduce perinatal transmission of the human immunodeficiency virus in developing countries. *New England Journal of Medicine*, 337(12), 853–856. doi:10.1056/nejm199709183371212.

Macklin, R. (1999). *Against relativism: Cultural diversity and the search for ethical universals in medicine*. New York: Oxford University Press.

Mahathir, M. (2013). *Telling it straight*. Singapore: Didier Millet Pte, Editions.

Mahdavi, P. (2008). *Passionate uprisings: Iran's sexual revolution*. Stanford, CA: Stanford University Press.

Mālik, A. Book 47, Number 47.1.8. *Al-Muwatta of Imam Malik ibn Anas: The first formulation of Islamic law*. http://ahadith.co.uk/chapter.php?cid=97 (Last accessed 23 August 2016).

Merican, M. I. (2000). Good clinical practice: Issues and challenges. *Medical Journal of Malaysia*, 55(2), 159–163.

Mir-Hosseini, Z. (2010). Sharia and national law in Iran. In J. M. Otto (Ed.). *Sharia incorporated: A comparative overview of the legal systems of twelve Muslim countries in past and present* (pp. 319–372). Leiden, The Netherlands: Leiden University Press.

Mir-Hosseini, Z. (2015). Muslim legal tradition and the challenge of gender equality. In Z. Mir-Hosseini, M. Al-Sharmani & J. Rumminger (Eds.). *Men in charge?: Rethinking authority in Muslim legal tradition* (pp. 13–40). London: Oneworld Publications.

Mir-Hosseini, Z., Al-Sharmani, M. & Rumminger, J. (Eds.). (2015). *Men in charge?: Rethinking authority in Muslim legal tradition*. London: Oneworld Publications.

Moazam, F. & Jafarey, A. M. (2005). Pakistan and biomedical ethics: Report from a Muslim country. *Cambridge Quarterly of Healthcare Ethics*, 14(03), 249–255.

Murphy, T. F. (2012). In defense of irreligious bioethics. *The American Journal of Bioethics*, 12(12), 3–10. doi:10.1080/15265161.2012.719262.

National Committee for Clinical Research (NCCR). (2016). National Committee for Clinical Research: Our purpose is to coordinate and encourage clinical trials in Malaysia. www.nccr.gov.my (Last accessed 20 August 2016).

Nuffield Council on Bioethics. (2002). *The ethics of research related to healthcare in developing countries*. London: Nuffield Council on Bioethics.

Nur, S. N. M. (2006). The ethics of human cloning: With reference to the Malaysian bioethical discourse (pp. 215–246). In H. Roetz (Ed.). *Cross-cultural issues in bioethics: The example of human cloning* (Vol. 27). Amsterdam, The Netherlands: Rodopi.

Office for Human Research Protections (OHRP). (2014). Office for Human Research Protections. www.hhs.gov/ohrp (Last accessed 1 December 2014).

Oguz, N. Y. (2003). Research ethics committees in developing countries and informed consent: With special reference to Turkey. *Journal of Laboratory and Clinical Medicine*, 141(5), 292–296.

Organisation of Islamic Cooperation. (2014). Organisation of Islamic Cooperation: The collective voice of the Muslim world. www.oic-oci.org (Last accessed 4 January 2014).

Oxford University Press. (2016). *Oxford English dictionary*. Online version. www.oed.com (Last accessed March 2016).

Padela, A. I. (2007). Islamic medical ethics: A primer. *Bioethics*, 21(3), 169–178.

Padela, A. I. (2013a). Islamic bioethics: Between sacred law, lived experiences, and state authority. *Theoretical Medicine and Bioethics*, 34(2), 65–80. doi:10.1007/s11017-013-9249-1.

Padela, A. I. (2013b). Islamic verdicts in health policy discourse: Porcine-based vaccines as a case study. *Zygon®*, 48(3), 655–670.

Padela, A. I. & Punekar, I. R. A. (2009). Emergency medical practice: Advancing cultural competence and reducing health care disparities. *Academic Emergency Medicine*, 16(1), 69–75. doi:10.1111/j.1553-2712.2008.00305.x.

Pakistan Medical & Dental Council. (2010). Code of Ethics. www.pmdc.org.pk/ethics. htm (Last accessed 20 March 2014).

Parker, M. (2012). *Ethical problems and genetics practice*. Cambridge: Cambridge University Press.

Pew Research Centre. (2015). The future of world religions: Population growth projections, 2010–2015. https://assets.pewresearch.org/wp-content/uploads/sites/11/2015/03/PF_15.04.02_ProjectionsFullReport.pdf (Last accessed 15 15 January 2020).

Pham, M. T., Rajić, A., Greig, J. D., Sargeant, J. M., Papadopoulos, A. & McEwen, S. A. (2014). A scoping review of scoping reviews: Advancing the approach and enhancing the consistency. *Research synthesis methods*, 5(4), 371–385.

Piedmont, R. L. & Village, A. (2009). *Research in the social scientific study of religion* (Vol. 20). Brill.

Plato (1914). *Plato: Euthyphro, Apology, Crito, Phaedo, Phaedrus* (H. N. Fowler, Trans.). Cambridge, MA: The Loeb Classical Library. Harvard University Press.

Pope, C., Ziebland, S. & Mays, N. (2000). Analysing qualitative data. *Bmj*, 320(7227), 114–116.

Rackham, H. (1952). *Aristotle* (Vol. 20). Cambridge, MA: The Loeb Classical Library. Harvard University Press.

Ramadan, T. (2009). *Radical reform: Islamic ethics and liberation*. New York: Oxford University Press.

Rathor, M. Y., Rani, M. F. A., Shah, A. S. B. M., Leman, W. I. B., Akter, S. F. U. & Omar, A. M. B. (2011). The principle of autonomy as related to personal decision making concerning health and research from an "Islamic viewpoint". *Journal of the Islamic Medical Association of North America*, 43(1). doi:10.5915/43-1-6396.

Raysūnī, A. (2005). *Imam al-Shatibi's theory of the higher objectives and intents of Islamic law*. London: International Institute of Islamic Thought.

Ritchie, J. & Lewis, J. (Eds.). (2003). *Qualitative research practice: A guide for social science students and researchers*. London: SAGE Publications.

Ryan, M. A. (2004). Beyond a Western bioethics? *Theological Studies*, 65(1), 158–177. doi:10.1177/004056390406500105.

Sachedina, A. (2006). No harm, no harassment: Major principles of health care ethics in Islam. In D. E. Guinn (Ed.). *Handbook of bioethics and religion* (pp. 265–290). Oxford University Press.

Sachedina, A. (2007). The search for Islamic bioethics principles. In R. E. Ashcroft, A. Dawson, H. Draper & J. McMillan (Eds.). *Principles of health care ethics* (pp. 117–126). Chichester, UK: John Wiley & Sons.

Sachedina, A. (2009). *Islamic biomedical ethics: Principles and application.* New York: Oxford University Press.

Sachedina, A. & Ainuddin, N. (2004). *Islamic biomedical ethics: Issues and resources.* Islamabad: COMSTECH.

Sahih Bukahri. Book 18, Hadith 1750. http://sunnah.com/riyadussaliheen/18/240 (Last accessed 19 August 2016).

Sahih Bukahri. Book 66, Hadith 49. http://sunnah.com/bukhari/66/49 (Last accessed 16 June 2016).

Sahih Muslim. Book 22, Hadith 133. https://sunnah.com/muslim/22/133 (Last accessed 5 November 2019).

Saleem, S. (2010). *Islam and women: Misconceptions and misperceptions.* Islamic Books.

Sandelowski, M. (1994). Focus on qualitative methods: The use of quotes in qualitative research. *Research in nursing & health*, 17(6), 479–482.

Sandelowski, M. (1998). Writing a good read: Strategies for re-presenting qualitative data. *Research in Nursing & Health*, 21(4), 375–382.

Sartell, E. & Padela, A. I. (2015). Adab and its significance for an Islamic medical ethics. *Journal of Medical Ethics*, 41(9), 756–761. doi:10.1136/medethics-2014-102276.

Setia, A. (2007). Three meanings of Islamic science: Toward operationalizing Islamization of science. *Islam and Science*, 5(1), 23–52.

Shabana, A. (2013). Religious and cultural legitimacy of bioethics: Lessons from Islamic bioethics. *Medicine, Health Care and Philosophy*, 16(4), 671–677. doi:10.1007/s11019-013-9472-6.

Shabana, A. (2014). Bioethics in Islamic thought. *Religion Compass*, 8(11), 337–346.

Shanawani, H. & Khalil, M.H. (2008). Reporting on "Islamic Bioethics" in the medical literature: Where are the experts? In J. Brockopp & T. Eich (Eds.). *Muslim medical ethics: From theory to practice* (pp. 213–228). University of South Carolina Press.

Shuaib, F. S. (2012). The Islamic legal system in Malaysia. *Pac. Rim L. & Pol'y J.*, 21, 85.

Siddiqui, A. (1997). Ethics in Islam: Key concepts and contemporary challenges. *Journal of Moral Education*, 26(4), 423–431. doi:10.1080/0305724970260403.

Silverman, D. (2013). *Doing qualitative research: A practical handbook* (4th ed.). Thousand Oaks, CA: SAGE Publications.

Silverman, H. (Ed.). (2017). *Research ethics in the Arab region.* Cham, Switzerland: Springer International Publishing.

Singer, P. (Ed.). (1994). *Ethics.* Oxford: Oxford University Press.

Sleem, H., El-Kamary, S. S. & Silverman, H. J. (2010). Identifying structures, processes, resources and needs of research ethics committees in Egypt. *BMC Medical Ethics*, 11(1). doi:10.1186/1472-6939-11-12.

Smith, D. J. (2004). Youth, sin and sex in Nigeria: Christianity and HIV/AIDS-related beliefs and behaviour among rural-urban migrants. *Culture, Health & Sexuality*, 6(5), 425–437.

Smith, J., Bekker, H. & Cheater, F. (2011). Theoretical versus pragmatic design in qualitative research. *Nurse Researcher*, 18(2), 39–51. doi:10.7748/nr2011.01.18.2.39.c8283.

Stake, R. (2000). Case studies. In N. Denzin & Y. Lincoln (Eds.). *Handbook of qualitative research* (2nd ed.) (pp. 435–454). Thousand Oaks, CA: SAGE.

Suleiman, A. B. & Merican, I. (2000). Research priorities: Future challenges. *Med J Malaysia*, 55(1), 1–6.

Suleman, M. (2016). Contributions and ambiguities in Islamic research ethics and research conducted in Muslim contexts: I – A thematic review of the literature. *Journal of Health and Culture* 1(1): 46–57.

Suleman, M. (2017). Biomedical research ethics in the Islamic context. Reflections on and challenges for Islamic bioethics. In A. Bagheri & K. A. Ali (Eds.). *Islamic bioethics: Current issues and challenges* (Vol. 2, 197–228). Singapore: World Scientific Publishing.

Syed, I. B. (1981). Islamic medicine: 1000 years ahead of its times. *Journal of the Islamic Medical Association of North America*, 13(1). doi:10.5915/13-1-11925.

Tan, A. K. G., Dunn, R. A., Samad, M. I. A. & Feisul, M. I. (2010). Sociodemographic and health-lifestyle determinants of obesity risks in Malaysia. *Asia-Pacific Journal of Public Health*, 23(2), 192–202. doi:10.1177/1010539509359535.

ten Have, H. (2013). Global bioethics: Transnational experiences and Islamic bioethics. *Zygon®*, 48(3), 600–617.

ten Have, H. & Gordijn, B. (2010). Travelling bioethics. *Medicine, Health Care and Philosophy*, 14(1), 1–3. doi:10.1007/s11019-010-9300-1.

The Holy Qur'an. Chapter 3, verse 104. http://corpus.quran.com/translation.jsp?chapter=3&verse=104 (Last accessed 28 December 2015).

The Holy Qur'an. Chapter 4, verse 34. http://corpus.quran.com/translation.jsp?chapter=4&verse=34 (Last accessed 2 March 2016).

The Holy Qur'an. Chapter 5, Verse 32. http://corpus.quran.com/translation.jsp?chapter=5&verse=32 (Last accessed 25 January 2014).

The Holy Qur'an. Chapter 16, verse 97. http://corpus.quran.com/translation.jsp?chapter=16&verse=97 (Last accessed 27 January 2014).

Tong, A., Sainsbury, P. & Craig, J. (2007). Consolidated criteria for reporting qualitative research (COREQ): A 32-item checklist for interviews and focus groups. *International Journal For Quality in Health Care*, 19(6), 349–357.

Tremayne, S. (2009). Law, ethics and donor technologies in Shia Iran. In D. Birenbaum-Carmeli & M. C. Inhorn, (Eds.). *Assisting reproduction, testing genes: Global encounters with the new Biotechnologies* (pp. 144–163). Oxford: Berghahn Books.

Von Denffer, A. (1983). *Ulum al Quran.* The Islamic Foundation.

Wadud, A. (1999). *Qur'an and woman: Re-reading the sacred text from a woman's perspective* (2nd ed.). New York: Oxford University Press.

Weindling, P. (2008). The Nazi medical experiments. In E. J. Emanuel (Ed.). *The Oxford textbook of clinical research ethics* (pp. 18–30). Oxford: Oxford University Press.

WHO (World Health Organisation). (2005). Islamic code of medical and health ethics. http://applications.emro.who.int/docs/EM_RC52_7_en.pdf (Last accessed 20 March 2014).

Widdershoven, G., Hope, T. & McMillan, J. (Eds.). (2008). *Empirical ethics in psychiatry (international perspectives in philosophy and psychiatry).* Oxford: Oxford University Press.

Winter, T. (Ed.). (2008). *The Cambridge companion to classical Islamic theology (Cambridge companions to religion)* (3rd ed.). Cambridge: Cambridge University Press.

Winter, T. J. & Williams, J. A. (2003). *Understanding Islam and the Muslims: Expanded to include the Muslim family and Islam and world peace.* Louisville, KY: Fons Vitae of Kentucky.

Yusuf, A. (2014). Ethical issues in research ethics governance and their application to the Malaysian context. DPhil thesis. University of Oxford.

Zahedi, F., Emami Razavi, S. H. & Larijani, B. (2009). A two-decade review of medical ethics in Iran. *Iranian J Publ Health*, 38(Suppl 1), 40–46.

Zahedi, F. & Larijani, B. (2008). National bioethical legislation and guidelines for biome-dical research in the Islamic Republic of Iran. *Bulletin of the World Health Organization*, 86(8), 630–634.

Zali, M. R., Shahraz, S. & Borzabadi, S. (2002). Bioethics in Iran: Legislation as the main problem. *Arch Iranian Med* 5(3), 136–140.

Index

abortion 130
abstinence 97, 98
accountability: legal and moral 128–136.
    See also moral accountability
advocacy 135–136
alcohol 76, 98
anxiety, moral 136–140
Arab states, and women/gender issues 119
Arabic translations, Greek virtue ethics 13
Ash'ari school 14–15, 102
atrocities 4–5, 9
authority 145–146, 198
autonomy 8, 69; and family 117–118,
    126; women's 111, 148–149; *see also*
    co-consent

Bangladeshi guidelines 70, 71
barrier contraception 80, 96, 129–130
benefits and risks 5, 78, 81, 85, 89, 91,
    101, 180, 197
bioethical discourse 79, 83–84, 89–92, 169
biomedical experts/researchers 85–88,
    94, 144–146, 147; advocacy role
    of 135–136; and personal faith/
    accountability 128–141, 149–151
breaches in ethical conduct 67, 69
bridge scholars 79, 83–85, 94, 144, 145
Brunei 67

capital punishment 107, 162
case study method 170–171
character 13, 69, 133
childbirth/maternity *see* women
Christianity 8, 14
CIOMS 33, 67, 68, 71, 199
co-consent 70–71, 111–121
Codes of Ethics 68
COHERD 4
community engagement, and scholars 81

condoms *see* barrier contraception
confidentiality 34, 180, 192
conscientious objection 130
consent: independent informed 5, 34–41,
    180; *see also* co-consent
conservatism, religious 85–86, 105–108
context, and universalism 9–10
contextual scholars 85–88, 94, 135, 144, 145
contraception 80, 96, 105, 112, 129–130
cooperation 145–146
culture 11–12, 120, 122, 152
custom (*urf*) 11–12, 17

data analysis 185–187, 196–198
death penalty 107, 162
deliberation *see* independent reasoning
depression 78
diversity 7–11
domestic violence 2–3, 122–124,
    136–140, 149
drug users, intravenous *see* IVDUs

embryo research 91–92; *see also* stem cells
empirical ethics 6–7
equality, gender 69, 119, 121
ethical analysis 191
ethical decision-making 17–21
ethical norms 6–7
ethical researchers, Muslim contexts 3
ethical review 180–181
ethical standards 5
ethico-legal edicts *see* legal edicts
ethics, Islamic 13–17
extramarital relationships 76, 80, 96, 98,
    102, 103, 162

family 149; and autonomy/consent
    117–118, 126; *see also* marriage; women
fatawah (legal edicts) *see* legal edicts

FIMA 97–98
foetal tissue 70; *see also* embryo research
framework approach 172
free will 14
freedom of religion 161
funding 4

gender issues *see* women
genetic manipulation 69
global health policy 108; on HIV/AIDS 95
governance mechanisms 3, 4–5; for
    breaches in ethical conduct 67, 69
Greek virtue ethics 13
guardian, male 111–112, 121, 122
Guardian Council, Iran 77, 166–168
Gulf Cooperation Council (GCC) 41

Hadith 13, 14–15, 86–87, 131–132, 147
health measures, disparity in 4
health research forums 4
Helsinki 68, 207
historical socioeconomic/religio-ethnic
    context: Iran 163–165; Malaysia
    156–160
HIV/AIDS research 4, 95–108, 146–147;
    ijtihad and fatawah to address 99–102;
    and *Maqasid/Maslaha* 102–105;
    personal faith/accountability and
    128–136; and religious conservatism
    105–108; variation in views 96–99
Hodgson, M. G. S. 11
homosexuality 96, 131, 162; *see also* LGBT
human rights *see* rights
husbands *see* co-consent

Ibn Sina 28, 169
ijtihad see independent reasoning
IKIM, Malaysia 89–90
Imam 165
independent reasoning 14, 15, 16, 18, 22,
    86–87, 90–91, 168; and HIV/AIDS
    99–102, 107
informed consent 34–41, 70
institutional review boards (IRBs),
    Malaysia 75
international guidelines 10; *see also*
    CIOMS; Helsinki; IOMS
international media, and HIV/AIDS
    research 105–106
interviews 169–172, 175–176,
    182–187
intimate partner violence *see*
    domestic violence
intuitive nature (*fitr'a*) 14, 132–133

IOMS 28, 71–72
Iran: centralised Islamic legal system
    77–78, 90, 91, 93; codes of ethics
    68; data collection in 176; on female
    consent 113–116; HIV/AIDS research
    105–108; national and regional ethical
    research committees 68; role of scholars
    in national guideline authorship 81–83;
    role of scholars in RECs and committees
    77–81; socioeconomic and religio-ethnic
    context 163–169
Islam: and culture(s) 11–12; and ethical
    decision-making 17–21; ethics 13–17;
    Islamic revival, Malaysia 158–160; in
    OIC guidelines 41, 67–69; origins
    12–13; *see also Qur'an*
"Islamic" guidelines 6
Islamic jurisprudence (*fiqh*) 16–17, 19, 90,
    92, 120
Islamic scholars 77–94, 143–144, 149, 192,
    195; bridge scholars and biomedical
    experts 79, 83–88; and guidelines 68–69,
    81–83; and HIV/AIDS research 98,
    102–105, 134–136, 146–147; in RECs
    and national committees 77–81; on
    women/gender issues 119–120
Islamicate 11–12
IVDUs, and HIV/AIDS research 95, 96,
    98–99, 102–105, 108, 135, 146–147

JAKIM 160, 161
Judaism 14

Khatami, President 167
Khomeini, Ayatollah 165–166
Kuwait guidelines 34

language, Islamic theology/law 145
Larijani, B. 68, 81, 168
Lebanon guidelines 34
legal edicts (*fatawah*) 22, 77, 86, 87,
    90, 144, 145, 168; and HIV/AIDS
    99–102, 107; Malaysia 162; motivation
    for seeking 92–93; on women/gender
    issues 70–71, 124
legal precedent, courts 86, 143
LGBT 96, 106–108, 131, 147, 162
limitations of the research 199–202
local communities, and principles/values 5, 9
local custom (*urf*) 11–12, 17

Macklin, R. 148
Malaysia: bridge scholars 83–85; data
    collection in 175–176; on female consent

113–116; HIV/AIDS research 102–108; multiculturalism 76, 79, 83, 162; and the OIC 28; parallel legal system 90–92, 158–162; RECs in 74; role of scholars in national guideline authorship 83; role of scholars in RECs and committees 79–81; socioeconomic and religio-ethnic context 156–163
Malaysian Medical Council (MMC) 75
Maqasid 15–16, 102–105, 134, 147
marginalised groups 69–70, 101, 106, 107, 121, 134; *see also* women
marriage 149; *see also* co-consent; domestic violence
maternity *see* pregnancy; women
MEHRC 75
migrant workers 67
MOHME 75, 169
moral accountability 92, 107, 142, 150–151; *see also* accountability
moral intuition 10
moral particularism 150, 152, 202
moral relativism 7–11, 148
moral virtues 13
muftis 162
Muhammad, the Prophet 12–13, 69, 114, 133
multiculturalism 76, 79, 162
Muslim context, in OIC guidelines 67–69
Muslim researchers 17–21, 23; *see also* biomedical experts/researchers
Muslim scholars *see* Islamic scholars
Muslims, population 2
Mu'tazili school 14–15, 102, 164

National Code of Ethics, Iran 169
National Committee of Medical Research Ethics 169
national councils, and Islamic ethico-legal issues 75–77
National Fatwah Council, Malaysia 80–81, 85, 87, 91, 161, 162
national guidelines, scholars' role in 81–83
NCCR 75
necessity 17
needle exchange programmes 85, 96, 99, 102–105, 108
NGOs 124
normative ethics 6–7
normative sources, Islamic 13–14, 86, 98, 99, 131–132, 143–144; *see also* *Hadith*; *Qur'an*

norms, contextual 12
Nuremberg Code 5

obedience (ta'ah) 119, 123–124, 140
objectivity 187
OIC/OIC countries: guideline review, findings 33–41; guideline review, methods 29–33; guidelines, protections **42–66**; mandate 28
oneness of God (tawhid) 132
organ transplantation 90
outsourcing 3, 156–157
oversight 5, 87

Padela, A. I. 11, 146
particularism/particularity 8–9, 150, 152, 202
permission *see* co-consent
personal experiences 75–77
personal faith values 128–141
Plato 14
porcine products 76, 85–86, 144, 186
pregnancy 70–71; *see also* women
presenting the data 198
professional values 97, 132, 133
protections, OIC guidelines **42–66**
public good 17, 78, 102–105, 134, 147
publication of data, and HIV/AIDS research 105–106

Qatar guidelines 34, 67, 70–71
qualitative methods 169–170, 182–185
questionnaires 182, 187–191, 193, 200
Qur'an 14–15, 86–87, 92; and ethico-moral thinking 131–133; ethics guidelines 69; primary source 13–14; on women/gender issues 69, 112–113, 118–121, 123–124, 140, 147, 149

rationality 102, 132
reason (aql) 132; *see also* independent reasoning
recruitment of participants 181–182
RECs: and HIV/AIDS research 106–107, 131; and the role of Islam/normative sources 75–87, 92–93
reflexivity 187, 193–195
relativism 7–11, 148
religio-cultural diversity 7–11; *see also* culture
reproductive issues 70–71, 100
research ethics guidelines *see* national guidelines; OIC/OIC countries
research instruments 182

revelation (*wahy*) 14–15, 132
revolution, Iran 165
rights: and biomedical experts 145; universal 148; women's 69, 124, 139–140
risks 5, 34; *see also* benefits and risks
Rouhani, President 167–168

sampling strategy for research participants 174–175
Saudi Arabia 28, 67
Saudi Arabian guidelines 34, 70–71
schools of theology (*kalam*) 14
semi-structured interviews *see* interviews
sex workers: health needs 80, 108; and HIV/AIDS research 105–108, 130–131
sexuality/sexual health 75, 76–77, 107, 125; *see also* HIV/AIDS research
Shariah (Islamic law) 10, 86, 146, 168; higher objectives 15–17; nationalised system, in Iran 90–91; parallel system, in Malaysia 90–92, 158–162; *see also* *Maqasid*; normative sources, Islamic
Shi'i: school of law 14–15; theocracy, Iran 164–165, 167–168
sin 92
social science researchers 96
stem cells 70, 79, 86, 91, 144
STIs (sexually transmitted diseases) 80; *see also* HIV/AIDS research
study visits 173

Sudan 41
Sunni, school of law 14–15
Supreme Leader, Iran 77, 165–166, 167, 168
sustainability 5, 6

totalitarianism 5
translation 181
transparency 145, 196

UAE guidelines 34–41, 67
Uganda 41
universalism 5, 7–11, 148, 202
urf 11–12, 17

vaccines 85–86, 144, 186
virtue ethics 16, 69

Wadud, A. 149
WHO 67, 122, 123
women 78, 110–126, 147–149; and autonomy/consent 70–71, 111–120; health/wellbeing, challenges to 121–126, 136–140; and OIC guidelines 68; in research 69–71, 82; sexuality/sexual health 125

yoga 78
young people 34, 80, 167

For Product Safety Concerns and Information please contact our EU
representative GPSR@taylorandfrancis.com
Taylor & Francis Verlag GmbH, Kaufingerstraße 24, 80331 München, Germany